Choose to be Healthy

Making Health Your #1 Priority

CHOOSE TO BE HEALTHY

Choose
to be
Healthy

Making Health Your #1 Priority

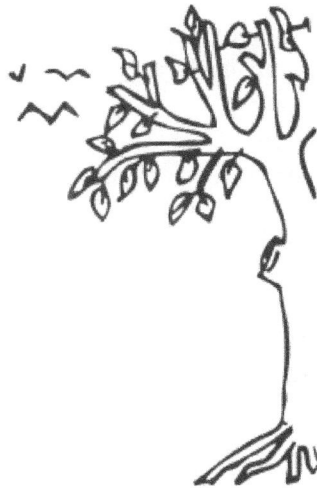

Janet Tayler MA, ND

CHOOSE TO BE HEALTHY

For more information, go to
www.Holistic-HealthPractice.com

First paperback edition 2020

ISBN 978-1-7331234-6-4

Cover design by: Andrew Kimbrell
Rival Signs Company, Weatherford, TX

Published by:

Legacy Lane Publishing
Weatherford, TX
www.LegacyLanePublishing.com

Acknowledgements

Thanks and gratitude to all my clients who have entrusted me with their health issues and invited me to be a part of their journeys over the years.

Thanks too to the many audience participants and friends who have asked the questions that form the body of this book … many of you are my dear Juice Plus family and business partners. I really value your support and belief in me.

My gratitude to Jay Martin and The Juice Plus+® Company for making my chosen career as a Naturopath that much easier and more effective. Your plant-based and wonderful products are central to my practice and have changed my own and so many other lives for the better.

I would not have started, let alone completed this book, without the expert and eagle-eyed guidance of Diane K. Bell of Legacy Lane Publishing. Thanks so very much for making your expertise available!

And to Garth, Sheba and Megan … thanks for your unconditional support and love … I am truly blessed to have you in my life!
2020

Dedication

I literally owe my life to my Mother - Florence "Paddy" Glover -
who passed peacefully to her next phase at 98 years young.
She was always an example and shining light to me:
from my earliest days of begrudgingly watering
flowers, fruit trees and vegetables in her abundant garden,
to being given my very own corner of the garden
(which to my excitement flourished as hers did,)
to slicing, dicing and preparing this home-grown produce,
cutting and arranging the many beautiful flowers,
drying herbs, canning fruit and vegetables,
and then smelling, tasting and finally eating our harvest.
This is where my Dad - Harold Glover - came in...
he loved nothing more than harvesting and sharing the bounty!
The two of them, by example, taught me the value and joy of
Honoring the Earth,
Looking to Nature for Health and Wellness and
Sharing these gifts with others
... and to my beloved husband Garth ...
Who has lovingly believed in me, supported my every effort
And been a willing guinea pig for my health advice and recipes!
This book honors you all.

Table of Contents

Introduction

My husband Garth and I immigrated to the United States from South Africa in 1995. While still living in a hotel, we were awe-struck by the loaded shelves in local grocery stores. As soon as we were in a position to prepare our own meals, I began buying the frozen, packaged and baked delicacies that had caught my eye. My early thoughts were: *this is food technology at its finest …* and *with the USDA as our watch-dog I don't have to worry!*

It took a year for both Garth and me to begin suffering with allergies, and colds and flu at the turn of every season. Bronchitis, with bouts of coughing that absolutely debilitated me, became the norm. Asthma, a childhood issue, returned full-bore. Even so, I did not go to a doctor for fear of "entering the system" and being prescribed anti-biotics or worse, steroids. I read up on herbal remedies and soothed the coughing with thyme, yarrow and mint tea; brought my fevers down with white willow bark and lemon tea and began adding supplements such as Echinacea and Goldenseal for acute illness; Spirulina, Evening Primrose oil, Vitamin C and multi-vitamins every day and Selenium, Zinc and digestive enzymes because someone at the health store recommended them. At one stage

1

we were buying around $350 of vitamins and other herbal supplements every month. I was literally throwing money down the drain … throwing good money after bad … spraying and praying for some sort of health relief which never came!

In 1999 I began studying for an ND (Doctor of Naturopathy.) The light bulb that went off nearly blinded me! Why had I not thought of nutrition as a way forward? Why had I only tried to fix symptoms?

Thankfully Garth was right behind me in clearing out all the brightly-colored packages, manufactured "food" and everything that contained questionable ingredients. We restocked with what we had eaten in South Africa … fresh fruit, vegetables, nuts, chicken, eggs, lamb and fish. We began to see some positive health changes … fewer allergy and sinus attacks and shorter colds-followed-by-bronchitis bouts.

We continued taking our supplements until another light bulb went off at an area wellness expo in 2001. The vendor next to me was a Juice Plus+® Partner. Over the 3-day expo, I read every brochure and research study she had and borrowed 3 videos to watch at home. The information turned our lives around. It was obvious to both of us that what we'd neglected to correct was our nutritional deficit. We realized that real, whole food was missing from our diets and that until this was restored, we would not regain our health. We began adding the available Juice Plus+® nutraceutical products (at that time fruit and vegetable capsules) to our cleaned-up diet. After finishing our supplements we did not replace them.

Within 6 short months I realized:

- ☺ I had not suffered another cold, flu, allergy or sinus attack.
- ☺ My nails were stronger and grew faster.
- ☺ I had not had a cold sore or mouth ulcer ... both frequent accessories before this!
- ☺ My skin looked younger and the puffy bags under my eyes disappeared.
- ☺ I was sleeping better and waking refreshed and energetic.
- ☺ The swelling and pain from arthritis in my hands had reduced.
- ☺ Best of all the bronchitis attacks had stopped.

Over time I have continued to see more health benefits from my lifestyle changes, namely:

- ☺ My hair is thicker and shinier.

☺ My dentist commented that I no longer had the early stages of gum disease … which had previously shown up as red marks around a bite of apple.

☺ I no longer bruise easily or dramatically (a disadvantage if I'm looking for sympathy after an injury!)

☺ After recent knee surgery (needed to repair an ancient injury) I had no bruising at all and the wound healed fast and clean.

☺ Another surprising change was reversing my bone density score from near osteopenia to healthy and strong bones.

☺ Neither Garth nor I take (or need) any medication. (Completing paperwork for annual medical check-ups takes no time at all!)

The media is filled with commentary about our escalating global health crisis. As such we are constantly bombarded with confusing and contradictory information. Flavor-of-the-month supplements and standard-of-care medications have become the norm. As a result it is really hard to steer a safe course. How confident are you that the latest recommendation is correct?

A helpful analogy may be: you are in a sailboat … the wind is gusting from first one direction and then another. You will bob and weave, be blown all over the place, take on water and even possibly capsize and drown … without a strong rudder.

This book … your rudder … will arm you with some:

- useful information
- good questions and answers
- tips to get you started
- some recipes to help you add more plant-based whole food
- recommended resources
- guidelines of where and how to start … taking back your health.

To this end, I have provided a shortened list of the many questions I've been asked at talks, presentations, seminars and in client consultations over the years. Questions on similar issues are divided into chapters. Both frequently asked questions (FAQs) and should be asked questions (SAQs) are included with the hope that my answers will give you insights and practical short cuts for your own health quest.

A word of warning: when "Just Googling It" … be aware that anyone can post on the internet and that opinions are just that.

CHOOSE TO BE HEALTHY

Search for supported, current, substantiated information and **become a critical thinker.** Cynicism can be a useful defense, but knowing what questions to ask and where to find reliable current information, will help you more.

I have recently heard of a great browser that does not track your searches, is unbiased and has total privacy ... called "DuckDuckGo." Rob Verkerk who writes for "What Doctors Don't Tell You" uses it, as he says, to "Detox from Google."

Taking control of your own and your family's health is the most important, exciting gift you can give.

Note:

The information provided in this book is intended to help readers play a more active role in their own health. It is not intended to replace the services and expertise of trained health professionals, particularly with regard to symptoms that may require diagnosis and/or immediate attention.

I wish you empowerment, vibrant health and longevity and with it more opportunity to dream!

Some ideas for using the book to best advantage:

- Read the questions in each chapter.
- Make notes on the blank page provided at the end of each chapter.
- Set up a "Master Mind" group with friends, associates or Juice Plus+® team and pool your ideas, thoughts and experiences for even greater impact.

1. **To set up a Master Mind group**, each participant buys a book.
2. The group leader decides the chapters or questions for consideration and
3. informs the group of what to read and what will be shared at each weekly meeting.
4. Meetings can be in a home, a coffee shop or via a Zoom conference call or change it up each time.
5. **Appendix C - "Daily Eating and Lifestyle Journal"** - on page 150 **may be copied free** to provide a daily journal outline. These may be shared as well ... insights about our personal health quests can be so helpful to those starting out on a take-healthy-back journey.
6. **Have fun and celebrate personal achievements!**

- Try the recipes ... make them your own!
- The appendices provide some information and some useful exercises to help you track your current health ... so you'll easily see where your focus needs to be.

♦ The resource section is limited to those books, videos and websites that I find most useful … they are just a start … <u>self-development is the name of the game here!</u>

<u>Questions Asked by Audiences and Clients</u>

Chapters 1 to 6

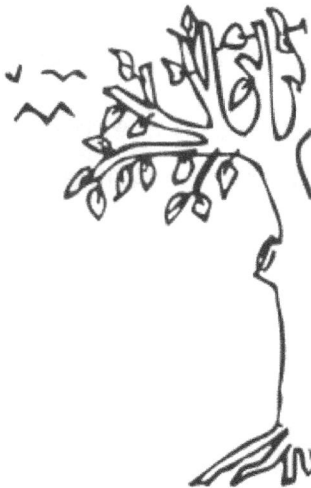

Chapter 1

Healthy Eating

> ➤ **What diet is the best?**

Ongoing research and personal experience suggests a plant-based diet is the most healthy. For me that also means it's the best. Preferably don't get hung up on the word "diet." As Michael Pollan aptly says:

> *"Eat whole food, not too much, mostly plants."*

> ➤ **Why is a plant-based diet the best?**

Thousands of research papers have concluded that the more plants we add to our diets, the healthier we become. Only plants provide the myriad phytonutrients (nutrients from plants) such as anti-oxidants, vitamins, minerals, soluble and insoluble fiber, trace minerals, phyto-estrogens and natural anti-inflammatories to name a few, that our bodies need to function efficiently and effectively every day.

CHOOSE TO BE HEALTHY

The **American Heart Association, American Diabetic Association** and **American Cancer Society** are all in favor of increasing fresh produce in the diet. Unfortunately, after all their combined campaigns to open the publics' eyes, the consumption of produce is nowhere near what it should be for good health. Researchers put this figure at 7-13 servings a day for the average working adult … and they do not regard ketchup, potato chips or fries as produce!

We evolved over a million years alongside thousands of plant species and were primarily gatherers and secondly hunters during all this time. There is a great deal of paleontological evidence that our daily food was bulbs, tubers, roots, fruit, berries, seeds and nuts (all in season). When our ancestors could, they caught and ate fish, birds, eggs and small animals. However, their diets were 80 to 90% plant-based and they thrived. Grains were not part of this early equation.

It is a misconception that only animals provide protein. There is protein in abundance in plants … for instance, broccoli has more protein than milk at 5.7g per cup; spinach, kale and Swiss chard have around 5g per cup. Nuts such as peanuts and almonds have around 6g per ounce. Quinoa needs a mention, weighing in at a hefty 6g per ¼C and containing all 9 essential amino acids. It is regarded as a "perfect" protein.

CHOOSE TO BE HEALTHY

Where most plants have little to no fat, some, such as avocados, edamame, olives, nuts and seeds provide healthy cholesterol-free fat: Omega 3s and both saturated and mono-unsaturated fats. These play a part in keeping our brains and heart and nerve cells functioning efficiently. I need to mention here that I'm **talking about whole plants** … not refined and processed plant oils like canola, soybean and peanut oils. **Please avoid these …along with partially- and fully-hydrogenated oils and margarines. They are NOT your friend!** Look for small bottles of organic coconut oil and organic unfiltered, first-pressed olive oil and use sparingly. A little goes a long way as fats and oils are calorie dense, but they are necessary for overall good health. For instance, the carotenoids and fat-soluble vitamins A and E must be eaten along with fat to be absorbed properly.

Let's take a quick look at one of Nature's constant processes: **oxidation**. As we breathe oxygen, we rust from inside out! Like the garden hose or wheelbarrow left outside all year … the hose becomes hard and inflexible and may rupture when the tap is turned on … while the strong metal wheelbarrow develops holes. The hose is your veins and arteries, the barrow your skin and organs. The process of oxidation ages us slowly causing damage, inflammation and eventual death. Sure it's going to happen, but who says we shouldn't slow it down if we can?

12

Nature provides plants with thousands of anti-oxidants so that they can withstand solar radiation, seasonal stressors, environmental and insect damage. When we eat plants, we in turn are provided with the same health-benefiting anti-oxidants … just another awesome reason to eat plants and lots of them.

Dr Bruce Ames tells us that not eating enough anti-oxidants every day is like standing unprotected in front of an x-ray machine!

Research shows us that we too can withstand these ravages just by adding more produce to our diets. Hence the global campaigns of *5-a-day*; *More Matters* and *Have a Plant*; the "Locavore" movement to eat more local, seasonal produce and products, and even the "Treat a Child" baskets of fruit provided free by many area grocers. By now every adult alive must know that fruit and veggies are good for us … they just don't know that they are so good they can save our lives!

If you still doubt that plants can provide your protein needs, think of the large herbivores: horses, antelopes, hippos, bison, elephants, rhinos and the great ape family. They are all longer-lived than their carnivore cousins, with better bone density and dental health. It is interesting to note that some parrots and giant tortoises live for between 80 and 100 years … on a purely plant-based diet.

(See http://gentleworld.org/10-protein-packed-plants/)

> ➤ **Is there anything I should know before adding more plants to my diet?**

No, not really! But let me give you some hints and tips anyway.

Be aware that when moving to a more plant-based diet you will need to eat more to get your energy needs. For example an iceberg lettuce side salad for lunch will have you racing for the candy vending machine within an hour of eating it! There are just too few nutrients to satisfy your needs. On the other hand, many vegetarians have weight and skin problems because they eat too much starch, sugar and fat (potatoes, rice, pasta, bread, cakes, cookies, candy etc) and few colorful, high-protein vegetables.

As Dr Mitra Ray, well-respected Microbiologist, says: *"Your brain loves pasta … it thrives on sugar* … **your will power depends on your blood sugar levels***"*

So when adapting to this healthy regimen, make sure your blood sugar remains level … if you're tiring, eat a piece of fruit, a handful of almonds or a square of cheese or some crudites. Be sure you **look for healthy alternatives before you get really hungry** … your brain will drive you to eat sugar to maintain its energy needs. Avoid fast or refined snacks. Check out the recipes for some very healthy alternatives in Chapter 9.

Drink water if you think you're hungry … you might be mistaking your body's thirst/hunger cues.

Some ideas for healthy, satisfying plant-based lunches and dinners are:

- Baked and stuffed squashes and mushrooms
- Filled baked potatoes or sweet potatoes
- Indian and Thai stir fries and curries
- Large mixed salads
- Mexican grilled vegetable fajitas
- Veggie, lentil and bean soups
- Italian vegetable lasagna
- Brown rice vegetable risottos
- Stuffed veggie or spring roll wraps.

CHOOSE TO BE HEALTHY

<u>Starting is easy if you're single</u>.

1. Just begin with one or more meatless meals or days a week and slowly work in more to give your tastes time to change.
2. Plan your weekly meals ... breakfasts, snacks, lunches and dinners. Print or write out easy recipes on a Sunday evening.
3. Don't buy too much fresh when you start out. You don't want to waste money by allowing unused food to spoil. Buy according to your weekly meal plan.
4. Be adventurous ... treat your taste buds. Remember to keep crunch in cooked veggies ... the closer to raw your food is, the faster you'll feel great. Feeling great will be motivation to continue.
5. Cut and chop a bag of veggies to use as crudités (raw) snacks. You can make or buy organic hummus, guacamole, Ranch and so on as dips. These veggies and a spoon of dip can be rolled into Ezekial tortillas or large Romaine lettuce leaves for a yummy snack.
6. Preferably start cooking simple meals 'from scratch.' Pre-cooked and packaged plant-based meals contain additives that you do not need. A piece of seasoned broiled, poached or blackened fish or chicken with a large mixed salad is easy, quick and delicious. Your body will love you.

7. Don't treat yourself with food. It's very easy to create cravings that way. If you want something you now regard as a poor choice, have some … but a smaller portion … and only after you've treated your body with something healthy! Treat yourself with an outing, a new outfit, or a bit of couch-potatoing … have fun while regaining your health … make it worth your while. You can even set up a special savings account and save the money you would normally pay out for over-the-counter meds, medications and supplements. Use it for a vacation.

8. As soon as you can, **eliminate sodas from your diet**. Sodas are directly-related to many health issues such as asthma, osteoporosis, obesity and diabetes to name a few. Instead drink filtered water, herbal teas (hot or cold) or Perrier water. The Greek word for water is *hydro* …so to *hydrate* means to drink water!

9. Initially you may feel you're missing the convenience of packaged foods. However, think about the incredible inconvenience, to say nothing of loss of time, income and life, if you don't take healthy back … and if instead, you become chronically ill.

10. Get a friend or family member to join you. There's **nothing better than an accountability buddy** and you'll accomplish more and really set your changes in stone with outside support.

CHOOSE TO BE HEALTHY

You have choices:

- ♦ to keep doing what you're currently doing
- ♦ to empower yourself, change and deliberately work on your health.

Einstein put it nicely when he said: *"The definition of insanity is doing something over and over again, expecting different results."*

If you don't change now ... where will your health be in say 5 years from now? Regret is one of the redundant feelings ... there's nothing you can do about it but wallow! Rather choose to steer your own healthy course ... starting now!

Here's a great idea from a wise and wiley Mom ...

****

IDEA

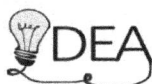

One Mom told me she placed paper baking cups in a muffin pan and filled them with tasty raw fruit and veg offerings ... strawberries, blueberries, carrot sticks, Clementine pieces, nuts, apple slices, broccoli and cauliflower florets, grapes, snap peas, celery sticks, an avocado dip and a homemade ranch dressing. She left the pan and a container of toothpicks out on the kitchen counter on a Saturday morning and when the kids, their friends or her hubby were in sight she casually helped herself to her choice. Not long and they were all tucking in. She didn't say a thing ... just acted natural ... so there was no negotiation needed and no objections to be overcome!

A wise woman indeed. ☺

****

CHOOSE TO BE HEALTHY

If you're in a relationship

1. Sit down and discuss your goals and reasons with your partner (and children.) Make sure they understand your motivation for change. It is especially important that your spouse doesn't sabotage your efforts by refusing to eat vegetables in front of the kids, or by making disparaging remarks about them. *Kids learn by example and by imitating the adults around them. They do as I do not as I say!* I have clients whose young husbands passed away far too early from heart disease. All were proudly "meat and potatoes" men and had stressful jobs.
2. The 10 tips for singles (above) apply to you too.
3. Make becoming healthy a game: set health goals; challenge your family to find exciting new healthy recipes for you to try together … or for them to make for you on your "day off!"
4. Check your kids' school subjects … they may already be learning about health and better choices. Get them to tell you what they learned, what they understood, how what they learned could help all of you. Let THEM teach YOU.
5. Make sure the grandparents understand and are on board with your efforts … they may unwittingly disrupt all your progress.
6. Dr Bill Sears says: *"Raise a grazer,"* meaning: encourage your kids to snack on healthy food between meals (like the muffin pan idea above.) The old rule of not eating

7. between meals causes especially active kids to eat too fast and too much at meal times. Sleep is inhibited after a large, undigested meal and obesity can result when too many calories are eaten and not used in activity. Eating habits are set in childhood and become really hard to correct in later years. On this score, the Anthropologist *Dr Margaret Meade said it is harder to change someone's eating habits than it is to change their religion!*

8. Eat at least one meal together each day, at a set table. Teach that smaller mouthfuls, chewed well, are better than gulping food down and leaving the table. Use this time to talk about each other's day. **Slow down.** Make mealtimes a celebration of time spent together, about laughing together, communicating and savoring healthy food.

9. Whatever you do **don't demand they change, don't make ultimatums or give up before you start. Be brav**e. Remember that Rome wasn't built in a day. **Persevere …your family health is worth it**.

10. I have a friend whose kids made a big thermometer and stuck it on the fridge. When the family stuck to her healthy menus and meals, they inked in a block for each day. When they reached agreed goals they took turns in choosing to do something special together.

11. You can DO this… you're strong … gaining and maintaining health is THE BEST cause in the world.

(Check out: **thesneakychef.com** and **forksoverknives.com**)

Chapter 1: Notes, Thoughts, Actions and Goals

Chapter 2

<u>Healthy Food Preparation</u>

> ➤ **How do I make vegetables as tasty as meat dishes?**

I love this question! Next time you cook meat, fish or chicken, try it without any fat, seasonings or sauces. I can almost bet you won't like it as much! **Seasonings and cooking methods are the key to success.** With all the seasonings and cooking methods available to us, no food need ever be bland and watery again.

I buy a variety of fresh produce once or twice a week and use dried and fresh herbs, lemon and lime juice and zest and vegetable <u>powders</u> (not salts): onion, garlic, cumin and <u>spices</u>: cardamom, chili, turmeric, ginger, cinnamon, clove, freshly ground black pepper, Himalayan salt and celery salt to add wonderful layered flavors to steamed, grilled, stir fried and baked veggies. A dab of organic unsalted butter, ghee or coconut oil just before serving adds extra richness and as I mentioned before, aids absorption of certain nutrients.

The only canned or frozen vegetables I use are artichokes, some beans and pasta sauces. I use frozen fruit almost every morning in smoothies. There are wonderful recipe books and entire websites devoted to vegetarian and vegan cuisines. I have included some of my favorites in the Resource section. For those of you who are adamantly carnivore ... no worries mate! Just try adding colorful veggies and fruit as often as possible. No-one need ever know!

> ➤ **My husband and kids hate boiled vegetables. How can I get them to eat more?**

Experiment with different cooking methods in your oven or on a stove-top:

❖ **Broiling ...** heat source is above and in the oven. Set food on a grid over a pan with a few tablespoons of water so that you don't burn and smoke your food. Keep an eye out ... food can catch quickly. Remember veggies are done in minutes this way.

❖ **Grilling ...** heat source is below ... use an outdoors grill or a cast-iron grill pan on the stove. Cook dry and then add sauces or seasonings later ... seasoning can burn ... this is how "blackened" fish or chicken are cooked

❖ **Roasting** ... dry heat at a constant temperature in an oven. This is a great method for hard root veggies and winter squashes, onions, peppers, etc. In a parchment-lined baking pan layer your choice of sliced or whole sweet potato, potato, butternut, acorn, Delicata squash or asparagus, eggplant, beets, parsnips, turnips, green beans ... you get the picture! Drizzle with olive or coconut oil, salt and fresh black pepper and/or any other herbs and spices that your little heart desires. Turn oven to 400F and roast for 20 minutes or until a toothpick indicates softness. Obviously whole root veggies and squashes will take longer (45 mins to an hour) and sliced or whole soft veggies less time (15 to 20 minutes). Checking for doneness won't injure the veggies, but may injure you ... be sure to use oven gloves!

❖ **Baking** ... cooks by using hot air and moisture in veggie quiches, fruit cobblers, cookies, cakes etc. Two hints here ... **DO use the recommended oven temperature and DO NOT check for doneness** until the recipe timing has been reached. Because you're dealing with air, your soufflé or spectacular cake will deflate before your very eyes if you open the oven to peek!

❖ **Toasting** ... either bake at 350 F, or use a low-heat broil ... Great for making granola, muesli, dessert or salad toppings ... place one or more of the following into a baking pan/sheet: rolled oats, sliced or broken nuts, sesame seeds, shredded unsweetened coconut, flax seeds. Use a metal spoon to keep the pan contents from catching and burning. When the nuts begin to brown, remove pan from oven and allow to cool at room temperature. Store in a Ziplock bag in the freezer, or in an airtight bottle till needed. **See recipes for muesli and granola in Chapter 9**.

❖ **Steaming ...** uses moist heat and cooks using steam from boiling water. Place a wooden or metal steamer over lightly boiling water ... **I add a 4 inch piece of fresh thyme, oregano, mint or rosemary to the boiling water for extra flavor.** Check for desired softness with a toothpick ... brighter color also indicates when cooked.

❖ **Sautéing (stir fry** with 1 T water and 1 T olive or coconut oil to prevent hydro-carbons forming ... the smoke and blackening caused by burning fat and sugars.) Veggie options are: cabbage, broccoli, cauliflower, carrots, spinach, kale, leek, onion, peppers, zucchini (aka courgette), celery, green beans, peas, etc... your pick. **Remember to choose as colorful as possible** ... this will ensure you're adding more plant servings and many more nutrients. Slice veggies and add small amounts at a time to the pan, keep stirring for a few minutes till just cooked ... keep in a warm bowl in the oven while stir frying the rest of the veggies. <u>Doing too much at one time will result in steamed veggies!</u>

❖ **Slow Cooking** ... in a "Crock Pot (ceramic pot inside an electric heater) is an easy and convenient way to make a casserole and more, while you are away at work or busy at home. The pot does the cooking for you ... no need to watch it. Read the instructions and you cannot go wrong!

❖ **Boiling** ... great for eggs, but not so great for veggies because it tends to kill off many nutrients. Baby potatoes are good boiled and drained ... then add butter or coconut oil, garlic powder, salt and black pepper for easy whole, mashed or smashed (lightly squashed!) garlic potatoes.

❖ **Better than boiling ... Blanch** veggies by pouring boiling water over sliced, room-temperature veggies such as tomatoes or nuts – to peel them easily – or over broccoli, zucchini, peas, asparagus, cauliflower and green beans, to slightly cook or "blanch" them. Drain well after about 5 minutes and season. Veggies like this are great for eating with dips, hummus, as starters and so on.

❖ **Poaching** ... also great for eggs ... place fish, chicken or sliced veggies in a pan with a lid and pour in just enough vegetable or chicken stock or vegetable milk to come halfway up the side of whatever you're poaching. I season the liquid with a little salt and herbs (for fish, chicken and veggies) or with spices, honey/sugar and a little red wine (for poached fruit … apples, pears and dried fruit.) The trick is to poach on a medium heat and keep "basting" – spooning over liquid to cook the upper side of the food as well. DO NOT turn the food as it becomes very tender and will break up easily. Chicken, fish and veggies done like this are great eaten as is, or diced and added to salads, pasta or grain dishes such as risottos.

❖ **Frying** … I never fry anything and I don't recommend you do either. Instead of French *fries* … try roasting chipped sweet potatoes, potatoes, beets and onions … all are delicious and much healthier! Hydro-carbons are created when frying food. These are highly oxidized food compounds that are injurious to health because they add to the free radical load in your cells. Furthermore, hot fat combined with carbohydrate (think French fries, fried pies, etc) creates another very toxic compound called acrylamide. Both deep frying and air-frying methods have been associated with hydro-carbon compounds and acrylamide formation. Both of these compounds are considered mutagenic, which means they can mutate your precious DNA. Think also of eating out … do you know for sure that deep fryers are cleaned out and old

rancid oil replaced with new clean oil? There are so many other healthy cooking methods to choose from, my take is: why take a chance with your health?
Don't get fried!

Chapter 2: Notes, Thoughts, Actions and Goals

Chapter 3

Health in General

> ➤ **What do you mean by "Whole" food?**

All produce is whole … whole produce is unprocessed or minimally processed … it has no ingredient list or nutrition labeling. It may have a cellophane wrapper (celery) or be in a plastic container (baby lettuce) but you recognize it as the whole/entire plant. Unpolished brown rice, lentils, dried beans (even when canned), quinoa, wheat berries, etc are all whole as long as husks have not been removed. If there is a label on grains, look for at least 2 to 3g of fiber per ¼ cup to know you're eating whole grain.

There are now little gold stick-on labels indicating *"100% whole grain"* on bakery in the USA. I suggest you still check the ingredient list and weed out products that have an excess of refined ingredients even if they're labeled as "whole" flour. Manufacturers have a nasty habit of trying to mask unhealthy, cheap and unnecessary filler ingredients with fancy labeling. Unleavened or flatbread is close to "whole," as are sprouted grain breads (*Ezekial* bread, tortillas and cereal spring to mind.)

Eggs in their shells are obviously whole. My opinion on whole eggs is this: they are a perfect food, just don't overdo consumption. They have a lot of cholesterol, but we need cholesterol for healthy brain function and research tells us an egg a day goes a long way to reduce depression in children and provides good levels of choline and sulphur which are needed to stave off multiple sclerosis and neurological damage.

Check that the eggs you buy are organic, that the hens have never been fed growth hormones or anti-biotics and have been entirely pasture-raised. Look for local small-farm producers. These eggs will be naturally high in Omega-3 because the hens eat insects out in their pastures … and insects have a high fat content. (Some African tribes thrive on the fat provided by roasted insects. Just thought you'd like to know!) For myself I definitely feel happy when looking at a nice sunny-side-up poached egg on a bed of spinach and kale with a side of diced mushrooms, tomato, peppers, cilantro and onions!

Make it a habit to 'shop the perimeter' of your local grocery stores. You will then be more likely to eat a clean and only whole food diet.

> ➢ **What chemicals should I be looking for in ingredient lists?**

That's a hard one to answer. Currently there are over 10,000 known "foodlike" substances in processed/manufactured food. **Please note, I said *"Foodlike"* ... but these are not food as our bodies know it!**

There are far too many out there to have been safety tested and too many coming onto the market as those in current use get a bad reputation! Here are a fraction of the chemicals commonly found in quantity, or residue, in common manufactured and farmed foods:

- ❦ those used as additives in high enough quantities to appear on ingredient lists (hydrogenated fats, *natamycin* ... an anti-fungal used as a preservative in products containing egg)
- ❦ those added as less than 2% of the total recipe - even if they are regarded as carcinogenic or mutagenic ... these do not have to be listed as ingredients and many have not yet been tested for safety in humans (azocarbonamide – a plasticizer in dough, nitrites and nitrates in smoked meat)
- ❦ those that leach into food via packaging (BHT)
- ❦ those that are used to spray crops (herbicide, fungicide, pesticide and waxes)

- ☞ those that are added to animal feed (growth hormones, antibiotics)
- ☞ those used in food production, such as detergents used to decaffeinate coffee and tea (methylene chloride)
- ☞ those used in the wine industry to color and flavor unripe grapes and clarify wine (mega-purple, isinglass, calcium chloride, added sugar)

Much of the industrial food complex does not have our best interests at heart. But times, as Bob Dylan said, they are a'changing ... and not too soon. Suffice to say, I recommend:

- ☙ moving away from processed food that isn't **clearly labeled. Choose food with as <u>few and recognizable ingredients</u> as possible**. If you don't think Great Grannie would have recognized an ingredient or added it to her recipe, it's probably not food as we know it.
- ☙ Feed your body real, whole food and you'll be on the right track. If your food is energetic, you will be too. Eat alive, not dead food! (Have you ever seen your carrots, potatoes and onions sprouting shoots or roots? That's because they're alive!)
- ☙ Be adventurous in trying new produce ... you may just discover a brand new favorite. Then check on the web for recipes ... have fun with it.
- ☙ Look for organic wherever possible, but remember that even organic produce can have pesticide, herbicide and fungicide residues, be ethylene irradiated (to give that

34

bright ripened look) and be waxed for longer shelf life. So carefully wash it all before devouring.

☙ Generally the "organic" label has been extremely hard won … these manufacturers are more likely to be honest about what's in their products.

☙ Don't be fooled by advertising and disclaimers. **Read ingredient labels as though your life depends on it** … it does! But don't become obsessive (like the young guy I saw at the grocery store … staring into a woman's cartload of party junk food and shaking his head, muttering that she should know better and that she was poisoning her kids! A man after my own heart I must admit. I caught his eye and grinned, nodding!) … just be alert to the contents of your own cart… and use the opportunity to hand out your Juice Plus+® business card!

☙ Eat produce in season and locally-grown whenever possible … it's more likely to be vine-ripened.

☙ Learn to cook from scratch … above all this skill will empower you and open your eyes to what REAL food is and how it should taste. Stretch yourself for your health.

☙ Take cooking lessons. Garth and I love joining a *Sur la Table* cooking class every now and then. We've met some awesome people. There are great cooking channel lessons and wonderful new and health-conscious foodie magazines and recipe books to choose from.

Give home-created spice rubs, chutneys, preserves, infused olive oil, etc for gifts. You never know, you may start a home-based business!

Take a look at Appendix A: "Weeding out the Sicko's" for some more useful dos and don'ts.

> **What do you mean by "Health?"**

I laughed when I saw that Joan Walsh (American journalist) said: *"A man's health can be judged on which he takes 2 at a time: pills or stairs!"* Short and sweet!

Wikipedia defines health as *a state of physical, mental and social well-being in which disease and infirmity are absent.*

I believe that health is more than just the absence of disease … in addition, for me it is the freedom to dream and realize your dreams; it encompasses spiritual and emotional well-being and spreads to the communities in which we live. When one of us is ill, the entire community suffers. When the community is healthy, even a newcomer is 'infused' as well.

To illustrate: A client of mine had felt ill and depressed for years. But doctors could find nothing wrong. After working diligently at an upgraded diet and a better sleep, exercise and relaxation regimen she was able to go on holiday with her grandchildren and enjoy being with them for the first time in

36

years. She cried as she told me how much she'd loved being around her kids and grandkids, how she'd had energy to play and had laughed and "come alive" again.

This is real health … everyone benefitted from one individual's better health and this created a spiral of better experiences. Her entire family was able to dream of more opportunities to share time together and make memories to keep long after the actual experience.

For me, **health is also a continuum**.

Go to **www.holistic-healthpractice.com**

and do the exercise under the "Circle of Life" tab to see where you are on the health continuum and to devise a plan for better health. I challenge you to track these goals (by journaling) for at least a week … better yet a month. Then celebrate your positive health changes.

> ➤ **Why is sleep so important for good health?**

Sleep is the time for metabolizing, regenerating, detoxifying and balancing. We have enough energy for one major process at a time. So, for instance, when you are running for your life (the fight or flight response,) your other systems shut down. Right then, all you need is for your heart to be beating and your muscles to be moving smoothly to help you escape. There is no time to stop and think, no time to talk, no time for digestion and your immune function goes on hold.

In today's stressful environment, sleep is the only time we have to lay down, really relax, recover and rebuild. By day we live in a fight or flight world from which it may seem there is no escape … we cannot fight or flee … we are trapped. So getting enough quality sleep is even more important than in your grandparents' time when life was slower.

The <u>benefits of 8 hours of uninterrupted sleep</u> are:

- ❧ waking up feeling energized and raring to go
- ❧ a clear mind
- ❧ healthy glowing skin
- ❧ no need for afternoon naps
- ❧ easy appetite and impulse control
- ❧ a fully functioning immune system
- ❧ a well detoxed brain and body
- ❧ a rested heart and relaxed vascular system.

So how do I achieve this you may ask?

CHOOSE TO BE HEALTHY

Here are 5 pre-sleep habits to develop:

1. Stop all blue light activities 2 hours before heading to bed (tv, cell phone, laptop, etc) and keep electronic devices out of the bedroom … think also electronic alarm clocks!
2. Stop eating 2 hours before bed to allow your stomach to empty. A cup of chamomile, peppermint or Red Bush (Rooibos) tea is great to aid digestion and begin to draw your energy down.
3. Set an alert for bedtime … and abide by it!
4. Have your bedroom as dark and quiet as possible … you may need an eye mask and ear plugs.
5. Use the 2 hours before bed to have a warm bath or shower; do some stretching, yoga or calming meditation to prepare your body for sleep.

If you're feeling sick … colds, flu, blocked sinuses, tummy upsets and more … please stay home and rest … better yet … get all the sleep you can! At these times your body needs to restore you to health and while you're running about being busy, your immune system will not be functioning efficiently … to say nothing of what you're spreading to those poor souls around you!

CHOOSE TO BE HEALTHY

To support your return to health …

- ✓ **Neti pots** are wonderful for sluicing the sinuses … it may sound less than pleasant, but it is soothing and a natural support to blocked sinuses. Make sure the water is only as warm as your wrist allows. Walmart, health stores and pharmacies sell both Neti pots **and packets of the saline powder** that goes into the water.
- ✓ We use *"Oscillococcinum"*… a homeopathic product, at the first sign of a cold. (Although these are really few and far between these days.)
- ✓ My daily go-to for immune support is the **trio of Juice Plus+® vegetable, fruit and berry capsules** and Juice Plus+® Omega Blend … 100% plant-sourced omegas. I never miss a day!

Good night … sleep tight!

Chapter 3: Notes, Thoughts, Actions and Goals

Chapter 4

About Specific Health Issues

> ➤ Why am I suddenly gluten-intolerant when I wasn't before?

To answer this one I'll have to take you on a quick hike through the history of bread-making.

Using whole grains for bread is a 10,000 year old tradition. Hard wheat berries were stored against insect and rat predation, in stone containers. As needed the berries would be hand stone-ground and the resulting "whole" flour would be used immediately to make flatbreads (pita, griddle cakes and so on.) Every meal would have included this bread ... healthy and minimally processed.

Come the industrial revolution, in 1870, the steel roller mill was invented. Millers could now separate the grains into component parts, removing nutrients like fiber and fat (the germ) which allowed for increased shelf life, greater distribution distances and a slew of new products. Thus whole brown rice became polished white rice, rice hulls, rice bran, rice syrup and puffed rice cereal, while whole winter wheat berries became refined flour, bread flour, wheat germ, wheat bran and so on. An added benefit was that insects and rats no longer recognized this refined and nutrient-deprived flour as a food source ... **now this should have made us stop and think!**

I see the gluten intolerance problem as twofold. Refining and the even newer technology: Genetic Modification (GM).

Refining: The original whole wheat berries had bran and wheat germ to balance out the small amount of natural gluten. Today's refined flours are almost pure gluten (wheat protein) and devoid of original nutrients. Because refining is a new creation (only 150 years old) our systems don't tolerate the resulting products well.

Genetic Modification: GM is much more insidious. Originally (1950's) it was touted as the savior that would eliminate world hunger by increasing the protein (gluten) content in wheat. The gene structure of wheat was tampered with to create a dwarf species, drought tolerant, able to thrive on synthetic fertilizers, resistant to pests, mold and herbicide. This resulted in wheat with very high gluten levels, but bathed in chemicals (herbicide, pesticide and fungicide) introduced into the genetic structure. What we have now doesn't resemble the mother wheat at all... and what we have now is almost epidemic levels of gut and neurological ill-health directly linked to this new "wheat." (Perhaps we should rename it "What?")

It is interesting that many of my clients are still able to eat non-GMO whole oats, kamut, rye and spelt without problems. These are the 'ancient' (heirloom) grains and related to original wheat.

All contain the original small amounts of gluten. However these same clients suffer bloating, diarrhea, headaches and gastric irritability almost immediately on eating most modern-day wheat products.

Note that **Celiac Disease is a highly dangerous auto-immune disease caused by an allergy to gluten**. It seems to run in families (this could be due to genetic disposition or to family eating habits.) The villi in the small intestine are destroyed, making it impossible to absorb nutrition. There is no cure as yet, but recognized early enough, sufferers can still thrive if they make a permanent change to a gluten-free and plant-based, whole food diet. In a way, those with celiac disease are lucky. The Gluten Intolerance Group estimates that 16% of Americans are gluten-sensitive whereas only 1% has been diagnosed with Celiac Disease. When enough intolerance is built up, celiac disease can result. I recommend that all my clients move towards a reduced or gluten-free diet. It's safer and healthier than the alternative. For a good text on gluten and its issues, read: "Wheat Belly" by Dr. William Davies.

> ➢ **What do I eat on a gluten-free diet?**

… pretty much anything that does not contain wheat, barley or rye, their flours and malt syrups. Be aware that even the communion wafers in church and the fillers, or actual capsules

****

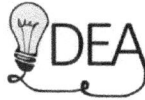

I had one client whose extremely swollen joints returned to normal and pain-free in under a month. Then she went to communion and had a major setback. It was she who alerted me to gluten or possible contamination in the wafers. Her church has since changed to brown rice wafers for its congregation.

****

used for medication, are probably wheat-based. Nowadays, although most people do not have Celiac Disease, they might suffer from ulcerative colitis or diverticulitis … they too feel better when they eliminate wheat products. Read "Idea" on the previous page for a real-life experience.

If you suffer from bloating, constipation, dizziness, headaches, achy swollen joints and/or diarrhea – try getting rid of wheat and journal how you're feeling. Chances are you'll be glad you did! The next question about Celiac Disease expands on gluten-free eating options for you.

➢ **I have Celiac Disease (CD) … what do you suggest I eat?**

If you are really committed to **making the following changes, you may go into remission** … which will feel like the CD has gone for good. However, eat gluten and your system will react violently. CD is apparently incurable … in other words your destroyed villi will not regrow. Maybe, maybe not … our bodies are miraculous when we understand and fully support their processes.

First thing is obviously to **eliminate gluten-containing products** from your pantry. This includes anything derived from wheat, barley, rye and triticale (a grain, laboratory-hybridized from wheat and rye). Even oats may be contaminated if it is processed on equipment that has processed a gluten grain! Next is to **read every ingredient label** to keep gluten out of your home. In addition, **work at healing your gut** by taking pre- and probiotics and **'getting rid of the whites'** (all refined food including flours, sugar, oils, pasta and rice.) Be aware that flour and starches (often from gluten grains) are used as thickeners in soups, yoghurts, puddings, custards, gravy … even ice-cream … **READ THOSE LABELS!**

Eat and do the following:

- ✓ Add a wide variety of fresh green and colored produce
- ✓ Drink water, green and herbal teas
- ✓ Reduce or stop eating at least farm-raised red meat. Farm-raising means animals are forced to eat grain which is not their natural diet. They are also highly stressed and the practice of using anti-biotics prophylactically causes even more problems. Eat only 100% pasture-raised meat (bison and venison are good choices.)
- ✓ Reduce alcohol and coffee. There are studies that show one glass of red wine with a meal and one cup of organic coffee a day, are beneficial to health. They add antioxidants; wine helps to destress and coffee clears brain fog. Be aware that too much of either is damaging to the liver and brain. Decaffeinated coffee is not a healthy option because detergents are used to defat coffee … the fat is where the caffeine resides … and detergent residues remain in the finished decaf coffee.

✓ Preferably eliminate cow's milk. Butter, ghee and hard cheeses made with natural enzymes and goat or sheep milk cheeses are okay (organic feta, cheddar, Gouda, Parmesan, etc) Many of the small organic cow's milk dairies sell their milk to big dairies who mix everything together ... so the advantage of organic milk is lost. Do your homework ...local raw, organic milk, from pasture-raised herds may be available to you.

✓ Eat 30 to 45g of fiber every day to help detoxify and clean out the colon ... beans, lentils, quinoa, brown rice, flax seeds, leafy greens, prunes, mangoes and blueberries all provide great plant protein as well as lots of fiber and minerals. All are needed for better gut health.

✓ Nowadays you will find shelves of gluten-free products at your grocers. Read ingredient lists and be careful not to substitute gluten for other harmful, unnecessary chemicals or too much sugar, salt and fat.

✓ If you enjoy chicken and fish, look for air-chilled, organic and pasture-raised chicken and eggs, and wild-caught ocean fish. The animal farm-raising practices leave much to be desired!

My go-to nutraceutical to help add extra bang for my nutritional buck is Juice Plus+® Fruit, Vegetable and Berry capsules and Juice Plus+® Complete smoothie powder. These 4 products will add 50 different gluten-free plants a day, flooding your system with the nutrients your body needs to heal and function effectively. Our family also takes Juice Plus+® Omegas – a 100% plant-sourced blend of omegas 3,5,6,7 and 9.

Juice Plus+® is available from Independent Partners. **www.taylers.juiceplus.com**

In addition, when making any lifestyle change, I recommend the following:

- Get 8 hours of sleep a night between 9.30pm and 8am
- Do at least 30 minutes of exercise a day.

These two components are particularly supportive because sleep will aid detoxification and calm your body, helping to keep you in balance as you change your lifestyle. Exercise helps to rev up your metabolism and again aids in digestion and detox through your liver, kidneys and skin.

- Drink plenty of filtered water to rehydrate and flush your detox organs as they go to work on your behalf. To work out the recommended amount for you: divide your current body weight in pounds by 2. The result, in ounces, is the water you need every day. (For example: You are 128 lbs …you need 64 oz …or 8 x 8oz glasses a day.)
- Make sure your friends and family know that you have CD; know that gluten is a poison for you and that real, whole food is what you have to eat to survive and thrive. You are welcome to make a copy of the relevant pages

about what you can eat. Your family especially may find the information helpful for when you visit for a meal! **Here's a tip: always be prepared to either take a gluten-free meal along as a table offering or eat clean before you go out.**

> ➤ **How many people survive a heart attack?**

The American Heart Association has been quoted as saying that 90% of first heart attacks are fatal! So the answer is, only 10%. In other words, the first sign of heart disease is death in 90% of cases … although the disease has been bubbling under for a long time.

Today emergency medicine is of enormous help in keeping people alive, but it cannot "out-medicate" a dangerous lifestyle. When the patient goes home, s/he will not survive long or live well without some relatively simple lifestyle changes. For my recommendations on the changes needed, reread the answer to the FAQ "What can I eat on a gluten-free diet?" The American Heart Association recommendations are similar. They are confident that heart disease is both avoidable and reversible when changing to a plant-based diet.

> ➤ **How can I tell if I'm a candidate for a heart attack?**

High blood pressure is one obvious symptom. Others include shortness of breath, headaches, radiating pain in the back and left side or down the arm. High levels of saturated (animal) fat, salt and sugar in the diet, lack of sleep, lack of cardio-vascular exercise, smoking and alcohol consumption are all risk behaviors. Heart disease is both avoidable and reversible, even if you are genetically predisposed.

(Watch **videos available on Netflix: "The Game Changers" and "Supersize Me."**)

> ➤ **How do you catch cancer?**

Cancer is not a disease you can "catch" … that is, it is not infectious. Cancer takes time to get started, relying on mutated genes within our DNA. When we eat poor food choices or overdo exercise we increase free radical damage to our cells. This basically means that our cells are bombarded by sparks that burn our delicate cells and the even more delicate DNA. When DNA gets damaged and cannot be repaired, a mutation might occur. When cells mutate they may begin to divide unnaturally fast … this could become a cancerous tumor.

Our bodies are amazing, however. At every turn, <u>if our immune systems are strong and fighting for us</u>, specialized cells hunt down and kill, eat or destroy cancer cells. So the most important thing you need to think about and do, is work towards optimal health as soon as possible. There is no specific "cancer diet." The best diet for health is a whole, plant-based diet with little to no refined anything ... especially sugar ... because it sets our organs, systems and processes up to function as they should.

Read the questions and answers about healthy eating in Chapter 1 ... they pertain to all the chronic diseases ... of which cancer is one.

➢ **What can I do to fight cancer?**

- I believe in a multi-pronged attack on cancer ... so,
- in addition to a clean, whole and plant-based diet
- stress reduction is very important.
- Good sleep patterns,
- healthy amounts of exercise,
- quiet times,
- drinking all the water you should,
- supporting detox with comforting Epsom salt and lavender baths all support good health.
- I further recommend colonics with a good colon therapist to detox the colon and help it rebuild its health and
- Reiki and Reflexology to balance energy and support the body's functions. These two therapies are particularly effective in the case of surgeries, when massage is best avoided.

- Fun and laughter are very important. There are actual "laughter clubs" in Japan. Their sole purpose is to promote better health and longevity through laughter.☺

- If you smoke, give up asap … if you don't, don't start! Avoid being around those who smoke …passive smoking is just as dangerous as lighting up yourself. Vaping is also injurious to your health. Your mucous membranes and lung tissue are highly sensitive … protect them from smoke, dust, particulate, fumes and temperature extremes.

- A chemical-free environment is important. Toxins in food and our work and home surroundings may exacerbate cancer and further depress the immune system. Think landscaping and herbicides or pesticides; Pest Control and pesticides or rat poison; Home Décor/Design and off-gassing of formaldehyde in drapes or furnishings, etc. (Both home owners and workmen will be exposed to these toxins.)

- Babies, small children and pets are particularly at risk from home-cleaning products because they are barefoot, crawling, even licking the surfaces. Substitute essential oils (EOs) such as lemon, orange, peppermint and oregano in water for potentially harmful products.

There is a relatively new field of study that shows we can turn our bad genes off and good genes on. It's called **Epigenetics**. (More about this later.) This is really good news because now we know we CAN do something to support ourselves and that we are not merely victims in the face of cancer. **Optimal nutrition which reduces oxidative stress and systemic inflammation is key to overcoming cancer.**

One of my clients is happy to share her experience in the hope that it may give you an idea of how to use both medical and naturopathic approaches, as she did. Let's call her Anne.

****

IDEA

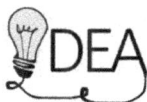

Anne met me at a gas station while we were filling up our cars. We got talking and she told me she had metastasized melanoma and had been given maybe 18 months to "get her papers in order." She had had surgery to remove the huge tumors, but had said no to chemotherapy and radiation. I offered her a free consult to review the natural therapies available to her.

We agreed on the following:

- ✓ *A weekly **Reiki** session to rebalance her energy.*
- ✓ *The same eating regimen recommended to those with CD (see above), except that she also decided to **cut out all dairy and red meat.***
- ✓ *That she **take two warm Epsom salts baths a day** … one in the morning, the second just before bed.*
- ✓ *She should get **8 to 10 hours of sleep a day**.*

- ✓ *She would **walk 15 to 20 minutes a day**. She also loved gardening, so continued to battle her weeds and do her **breathing exercises** outside in the fresh air.*
- ✓ *She was taking handfuls of supplements each day ... we reviewed these and eliminated about 75% of them.*
- ✓ *We agreed on 5 **daily affirmations** specific to her needs.*
- ✓ *I made up a **calming EO spritz** for her to use before bed or whenever she felt anxious.*
- ✓ *She added the **trio of Juice Plus+® Fruit, Vegetable and Berry capsules** to her daily regimen ... but instead of 2 of each a day, she opted to take 4 a day, or even 6 when she'd had a rough day, or was feeling a cold coming on.*
- ✓ *She **listened to soft, Baroque music** on most days; she read her Bible and other spiritually-supportive books; she only watched a few hours of TV a day ... no news or politics! She said if something bad was happening there was nothing she could do about it anyway ... that she wanted to stay upbeat!*

After a month, her scars had healed well. The discoloration and inflammation around them had disappeared. After another month she no longer got colds and decided against

56

having the recommended flu and shingles vaccinations. Her oncologist was really happy with her bloodwork and agreed to support her lifestyle efforts although he told her he was worried about some of her decisions.

18 months came and went nearly 11 years ago. Anne is still very conscious about maintaining the changes she put into place. She is now nearly 80 and her doctors are satisfied that what she's doing is exactly what she should be doing.

****

CHOOSE TO BE HEALTHY

> ➢ **Why is obesity dangerous?**

One of the gravest dangers of obesity is Metabolic Syndrome, which is the precursor of Type II Diabetes.

In one respect knowing you have a diagnosis of Metabolic Syndrome is hugely positive … you do not yet have Type II Diabetes … you still have the opportunity to fully regain your health. You can regain your health as long as you lose weight and balance your blood sugar ASAP.

I recommend following the Celiac Disease lifestyle, laid out in Chapter 4, to all my over-weight and obese clients. I don't believe in beating about the bush. We all know when we're carrying weight and the media is full of the health issues caused by obesity, including: heart disease, depression, cancer, joint and spinal injuries, depressed immunity, rampant systemic inflammation resulting in gout, arthritis and skin issues. Obesity is causing our kiddos to have heart disease and become Type II diabetic! Type II used to be called "Adult onset diabetes." No longer! Children as young as 8 have full-blown Type II diabetes. Early obesity can be an early death sentence. This is NOT an issue of body shaming … it is a question of having the life and health that is our birthright.

It is statistics like this, that cause **Dr Katz of the Yale-Griffin Prevention Research Center to predict that:** *"This generation of children will be the first to pre-decease its parents!"*

An important fact in taming weight gain is: whenever you eat a high-calorie meal ... in fact anything more than about 500 calories ... whatever your body doesn't use within an hour or two is converted straight to fat and stored. Each meal and snack should be carefully considered so that storage is stopped. Exercise uses calories, but not as many as you'd hope ... Google it (or try out "DuckDuckGo" browser) and see for yourself.

"Eat to live, don't live to eat."

"Eat only nutrient-dense food"

"Eliminate calorie-high, nutrient-deficient choices."

> ➤ **I don't want to diet, so how can I help my family be more healthy?**

The *Shred 10 Program* is perfect for resetting, detoxifying and calming an over-active system. It is not per se a weight reduction program, but when continued for longer than 10 days, it will help to re-educate the palate, coach about better food choices and help the participant follow a better health path than the one which caused them to gain weight in the first place.

My husband and I have done the *Shred 10* at least once a month for about two years. It's easy to stay the course for 10 days; we find we lose inches in the right places; we feel energetic and become more conscious of rehydrating, exercising and sleeping properly. It gently resets our course. It's said we all need at least 7 repetitions before we make a habit of a new activity … and it's so easy to be blown off course!

The program, which is perfect for the whole family, entails the following **10 daily additions or eliminations**:

1. Drinking a **Juice Plus+® Complete smoothie** for breakfast and again for supper.
2. Eating a **healthy fresh and raw-loaded salad** … which may include fish or chicken … for lunch. If a snack is needed mid-morning or mid-afternoon, a piece of fruit or a Juice Plus+® Complete snack bar is good.
3. **Eliminating all added sugar and gluten,**
4. **Eliminating caffeine and alcohol.**
5. Eliminating red meat,
6. **Drinking at least 8 glasses of filtered water** every day.
7. No more **eating after 6.30pm**
8. Going to **sleep by 10pm … for at least 8 hours.**
9. Doing cardio-vascular exercise for at least 30 minutes a day.
10. Taking **2 of each of the Juice Plus+® "quad" of capsules**: Vegetable, Fruit, Berry and Omega Blend with a large glass of water every day.

Looks exactly like my recommendations for heart issues, cancer, CD, diabetes and so on, doesn't it?

CHOOSE TO BE HEALTHY

Are you getting the picture?

Most of the **so-called chronic diseases of our time can be considered symptoms of our poor lifestyle choices** … hence the title and contents of this book:

"Choose to be Healthy."

You truly DO HAVE THE CHOICE. YOU CAN TAKE HEALTHY BACK. Isn't it worth it?

> ➢ **Can anything be done about Alzheimer's Disease (AD)?**

Alzheimer's is definitely the scourge of the century. Currently in 2019, there are 5 million people diagnosed with AD, with the prediction of 14 million by 2050. It is the leading cause of death worldwide. AD is being called *Type III Diabetes*. This is because there seems to be a component of poor sugar metabolism, or Metabolic Syndrome associated with AD.

What we know about AD is that two types of sticky proteins (called Amyloid plaques and Tare tangles) glue up the neurons of the brain, slowing down and stopping the essential nerve signals that are needed for every single process or thought or action that we do.

A research study published in the New Scientist in January 2019, proposes that these plaques and tangles may actually be the body's best defense against bacteria that have crossed the blood-brain barrier. The theory goes: Gum disease is a known risk factor, and the gingivitis bacteria (*Porphyromonas Gingivalis*) is known to produce two enzymes that can feed on and inflame brain tissue if it gets into the bloodstream and from there into the brain itself. The injured brain tissue forms plaques to protect itself from further bacterial damage.

Knowing these different theories helps us in this way:

- We need to practice good oral hygiene. A good friend of mine and dentist of note recommends we "FBI" ... **Floss, Brush, Irrigate** ... in that order ... twice a day, or even after every meal. Avoid mouth washes that strip away good bacteria from your mouth. A healthier alternative is a single drop of oregano, lemon or peppermint EO in a little water.
- **Eliminate refined and added sugar, sodas, sugary candy**. Review the question about how to avoid diabetes, on pg. 58 and the Celiac Disease food options on pg. 46 .
- **Reduce systemic inflammation and oxidation** with clean, whole food and conscious healthy eating.
- Because Juice Plus+® has been shown to consistently reduce *homocysteine* and *C-Reactive Protein (CRP)* in research studies and because research also tells us that increased levels of these are associated with AD, **adding Juice Plus+® Vegetable, Fruit and Berry capsules makes good sense.**

- <u>Healthline.com</u> expands on recent research showing how Omega 3 in particular improves memory, alertness, depression, anxiety and learning in humans. Juice Plus+® Omega Blend is 100% plant-based, thereby avoiding the "fishy burp" and potential heavy-metal issues linked with fish liver oils. *Nordic Naturals* and *Carlsons* also produce high-grade Krill oil … another good source of Omega 3.

In addition, for all the reasons noted before …

- Continue to get daily **cardio-vascular exercise** for as long as possible.
- Drink the **recommended amount of water** every day.
- Get the **recommended sleep** every day.
- **Stay connected with positive, fun people**.
- Get **brain exercise**: do puzzles, learn new things, read … keep those neurons sparking!
- **Buy all your medications from the same pharmacist**, so that s/he can constantly monitor and review drug interactions on your behalf. Many of my clients have been able to reduce unnecessary medications by asking for this service. **Over-medication or medication inter-actions or side effects are possible causes of so-called dementia**.
- Ask your doctor to help you reduce medication by monitoring your health markers. Tell him or her about the lifestyle changes you're making. Remember that **Juice**

Plus+® is like a salad bar in a capsule. It is whole food … not a supplement, and is the most thoroughly researched nutrition product ever. Ask your Juice Plus+® Partner to give you information to show your doctor, so that he understands what you're taking.

> ➤ **Can I do anything for my child who has autism?**

Absolutely yes!

As with any brain-related issues such as Autism, Attention Deficit Disorder (ADD,) Attention Deficit Hyperactivity Disorder (ADHD,) Obsessive Compulsive Disorder (OCD), epilepsy, dementias and even genetic disabilities such as Downs Syndrome … nutrition should be the first port of call.

Dr Bill Sears talks about **Nutrition Deficit Disorder** (NDD) as the new health frontier for children. This is a must-buy book for any parent dealing with any of these health concerns.

Follow the same guidelines for **firstly cleaning up your child's diet and then adding only supportive whole and healthy food choices** as outlined in previous questions above.

Specific dietary needs are:

- ☙ Eliminate gluten and dairy ASAP. Nowadays most children range from sensitive to highly sensitive, to these foods. Furthermore, as gluten and dairy are digested they break down into peptides that mimic opiate drugs and are highly addictive. Be aware that elimination will cause actual withdrawal symptoms. Persevere with elimination and the gut will begin to heal.

- Eliminate all food dyes/coloring, artificial sweeteners, MSG (a toxic flavorant) and preservatives … preferably blend your own fresh fruit and veggies … a mix of raw and cooked

- Omega 3's found in: wild-caught salmon and other oily fish (such as pilchards, sardines and cod), whole pasture-raised eggs and chicken.

- Juice Plus+® Omega Blend is 100% plant-based and an excellent option.

- Juice Plus+® Chewables will provide dense nutrition, wonderful anti-oxidant support and digestion-supporting fiber. If your child has trouble chewing and swallowing the gummies, melt 2 of each color in half a glass of warm water … drink in the morning. Over time many children graduate to chewing the gummies instead.

- In addition consult with your Pediatrician about a recommended Pro-biotic and maybe Digestive Enzyme blend to further support gut health and digestion. Children with autism often have issues with taste and texture as well. You will need to go really slowly when changing diet or adding in new options. Be gently persistent … your patience will be rewarded in sweet and unexpected ways.

A young client of mine called me one evening crying as she told me her autistic youngster had made eye contact with her for the first time. Something we take so for granted had been a major milestone in the development of her son. He continues to make progress on the regimen her Pediatrician and I recommended and is now able to remain in school and functions better.

A good resource book and guide is: "Naturally Healing Autism: the Complete Step-by-step Resource Handbook for Parents," by Karen Thomas (2015) who reversed her own son's autism.

A word about **Downs Syndrome kiddos** … These angelic children have a genetic disorder which may involve gastro-intestinal and/or heart issues and problems with obesity and therefore diabetes.

Again, even though the condition is irreversible, the answer is to clean up the diet … removing flavorants, refined products, colorants, artificial and unnecessary chemicals … and supporting children's health and wellbeing with whole, plant-based food, exercise, plenty of water, occupational therapy, fun activities and restorative sleep.

Chapter 4: Notes, Thoughts, Actions and Goals

Chapter 5

<u>Health and Exercise</u>

> ➤ **Which should I start with ... exercise or diet?**

Whoever first said: *"You cannot out-exercise a poor diet,"* said it right!

When you begin with the fuel you give your body every day, you will benefit by sleeping better, recovering and healing faster and generally feeling more alive. When that happens you will want to exercise ... which means you'll be in a better position to choose the exercise that's right for you ... the one you will <u>want to do, consistently, every day</u>. Only then will exercise actually benefit your body.

Exercise can be extremely destructive. It can leave you with sprains, torn muscles, joint injuries, open to infection and more. **Fueling for great performance** is one thing, but many athletes forget **to fuel for recovery** as well. This is why high-level athletes need much more food than your average Joe. It's fuel for both their performance and recovery. But it's **not just quantity of food** that's at issue ... **quality of food** is even more important. Current sport research suggests high-level athletes eat 9 to 15 servings of fresh produce every day. Let's see why this is.

CHOOSE TO BE HEALTHY

We all breathe oxygen which causes us to be oxidized slowly throughout our lives. When we exercise, this process speeds up … because we breathe faster (more oxygen causes more oxidation.) In addition, refined and sugary, fatty and junk foods create their own havoc by increasing oxidative damage.

In order to reduce oxidative damage we have to consume large amounts of anti-oxidants. **One anti-oxidant quenches one free radical**. Free radicals are oxidation agents. They are literally sparks that burn where they touch our cells or DNA, millions of times a day, causing untold damage. Over time our bodies may not have the capability, or enough fuel, to repair damage. This is how chronic conditions set up.

Think about a top racehorse. If you owned one would you feed it junk or just anything you could lay your hands on? I'm betting that you'd study its needs and make absolutely sure you provided for them!

There's an apt quote by Chungliang Al Huang (Taoist Philosopher)

> *"Many people treat their bodies as if they were rented from Hertz – something they use to get around in, but nothing they really care about understanding."*

Let me tell you my story … to illustrate that even with a bad start, you can still choose to become healthy!

****

IDEA

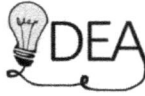

As a Physical Education student I lived in a university dorm. I ate more chocolate, bread and overcooked vegetables (and drank more coffee and alcohol) than at any time in my life. I was your proverbial Energizer Bunny! Because I was always on the go ... playing every sport imaginable ... I was also always hungry.

Over four years I sustained muscle tears, joint sprains, multiple upper-respiratory infections, 2 fractures and in one gymnastics accident, ripped the medial and cruciate ligaments and cartilage in my right knee. This was all too much for my body to repair alone. I was set up for chronic inflammation in many of my joints. It was never suggested that I change my diet or even that diet was my major problem. I believed that I could out-exercise my hideous diet ... and boy was I wrong!

Forty years on, I've had another major knee surgery to repair wear and tear on the same knee, but already the outcome is better. The scar and joint has healed incredibly fast and clean and 6 months after surgery I'm already much more mobile and pain-free than I have been in years.

So what was the difference?

I am in no doubt that it's my changed lifestyle ... in particular a diet that now fuels for both everyday performance and recovery:

- ✓ *A clean, plant-based diet with some eggs, fish and chicken*
- ✓ *Daily, 30 minutes to 1 hour of exercise*
- ✓ *8 hours of sleep a night*
- ✓ *Water to rehydrate*
- ✓ *Juice Plus+® as my daily food addition*

****

> ➤ **Is there any time we shouldn't exercise?**

If you've ever been near the critical care unit of a hospital you'll know the answer to that question is "NO!"

Even fully comatose and quadriplegic patients of all ages get twice daily workouts. If they didn't, their muscles would atrophy and they would fade away. Look at babies ... they move continuously from birth. In fact even fetuses swim about for 9 months!

Our body's energy is made by mitochondria ... tiny organelles within almost every cell. Muscle and liver cells have the most. An interesting fact is that as we do more exercise, our bodies produce more mitochondria in the muscle cells ... as we stop exercising, mitochondrial numbers decrease. A literal case of **"use them or lose them!"** If you start an exercise program, chances are you'll feel exhausted for a time, and then slowly you'll become more and more fit as mitochondria are added to support your increased energy needs. Stick with the program ... you will benefit so much!

Dr. Mitra Ray (Cell Biologist) tells us that we should exercise all the cells that are not injured or sick ... to tell the body that we still need them!

I recently had major knee surgery and discovered that Dr Ray is compassionate! The Physical Therapist in the hospital exercised even my extremely injured and painful knee **immediately after**

surgery! If I'd been less than comatose I may have tried to escape! In retrospect, I have to admit that I would not have done the exercises on my own. The PTs knew better and I'm so thankful now that they didn't give me a choice or ask for my opinion. I have recovered so much faster because of the twice daily exercises. Suffice to say, exercise is critical to life.

➢ **What is the best form of exercise?**

The exercise you will do consistently is the best exercise for you.

However, **cardio-vascular exercise supports our bodies best**, because it builds and tones the heart (cardio,) all the vessels (vascular) and all the muscles. Swimming, walking and dancing are wonderful for those who don't like to run.

"Exercise" is movement … so gardening, house-cleaning, walking to and from your car in a parking lot, climbing up and down stairs at work, walking your dog, tearing after your baby or grandchild and so on, are all forms of exercise too. If you have a "Fit Bit" or similar device, you'll know that steps are steps … it doesn't matter where you do them, it matters that you DO them!

The **hidden gifts of exercise** are that it raises endorphin levels … the so-called "runner's high" … reduces excess stress hormones and supports better sleep habits ... yet more benefit in our stressed-out lives.

Chapter 5: Notes, Thoughts, Actions and Goals

Chapter 6

Cleansing and Detoxification

> ➤ **What do you think about fasting?**

Fasting can be really helpful when done correctly. My Mom had a 1- or 2-day water and raw fruit and/or leafy salad-fast every month for as long as I can remember. She passed away at 98 taking no medications and living a really healthy lifestyle traveling and having fun until the end. If you are already relatively healthy, this type of fast can only benefit you.

The *Shred 10* **program** (in Chapter 4) is slow and supportive enough for most constitutions … and a very doable 10 days. I have many friends and clients who have used the program for monthly cleanses, on-going lifestyle change and one-off fasts to feel-good-quick and get-into-the bridal-gown. All have had great results.

Juice fasts are wonderful … make sure you juice more greens than fruit … fruit is high in sugar and needs to be diluted with water or reduced by lots of veggie protein and fiber. Dr Humbart Santillo has a few juice combination options to benefit the different organs. (*"Your Body Speaks, Your Body Heals."*)

For instance: **liver** – carrot, apple, dandelion greens; **kidneys** – carrot, parsley, apple; **bowel** – spinach, apple, carrot. Notice how carrots and apples are broadly beneficial to digestive health.

Personally I prefer using my *Vitamix* and retaining all the cellulose, to using a juicer that separates out the cellulose and some fiber.

In either case, **remember that when vegetables are macerated in a high-speed blender, chopped or grated, more nutrients become available to us. This is also why chewing our food well is so important.**

There is a great **all-vegetable soup you can try for a 3-day cleanse** … use the Bean and Vegetable recipe in Chapter 9 - just leave out all the beans and olive oil in the recipe for this fast. Have 1 to 2 bowls of soup for every meal and 1 bowl for a snack. In other words … this is all you eat for 3 days, morning, noon and night. It's soothing, calming to an inflamed digestive system and gently detoxing. You may also drink hot Rooibos, chamomile or Peppermint teas and water with or without lemon/lime.

I have done this soup cleanse starting on a Friday and ending on a Sunday. Start eating light meals again on the fourth day … easing back slowly into your usual healthy routine.

If you are depleted because of chronic illness or obesity, chances are your organs will need some extra support. It will be best to start slowly, giving your body a chance to get accustomed to the changes. Do not attempt to reduce organic overload overnight! There is no silver bullet to detoxification … what went into you over the years will have to come out at a pace that your body can support. Too fast and you could be further weakened.

You might want to treat yourself to a health spa where you will detox under constant medical supervision. Another option is to have a series of colonics at a certified clinic. Colonics work extremely well to gently remove accumulated mucus and waste from the bowel.

Whatever you decide, **be patient and compassionate with yourself, but get started**.

No matter what cleanse or fast you decide to do, make sure you get enough rest; drink lots of water; avoid all animal products, stimulants and sedatives; add Juice Plus+® capsules or Chewables for extra anti-oxidant support and take a multi-organism probiotic for added digestive benefit.

> ➢ **Why do you say that the skin is an organ?**

This question is relevant from a Naturopath's viewpoint, because clean, well-nourished and undamaged skin is your best first defense against infection and invasion. The condition of visible skin, among other things, is one aid that helps me decide how best to support my clients' health.

One definition of an organ is: *A part of an organism that is typically self-contained and has a specific vital function, such as the heart or liver in humans.* Another adds ...*an organ is a collection of tissues which have a common function.*

- ✓ The vital functions your skin performs are: **excretion** via the sebaceous glands and sweat pores which help to reduce your body's toxic load; **protection** … it totally self-contains you and its acid mantle (or barrier) helps to kill microbes that land on your skin and keep out harmful chemicals; it **regulates your temperature** by sweating and shivering - it literally stops you evaporating to death! It **waterproofs** you; it **keeps your brain in touch with your outer world** 24-7 … via thousands of nerve sensors; it allows for **free and supple movement**; it **provides cushioning** from knocks and falls; Melanin **protects** against the sun's UV-rays … more melanin produces darker skin, less results in fair skin; your skin **makes Vitamin D** … needed to convert calcium into bone.
- ✓ Your skin is a part of you … "the organism."
- ✓ An adult has 8 lbs of skin which spreads out to 22 square feet (2 square meters.)
- ✓ It takes roughly 5 weeks for totally new skin cells to work their way to the surface. (Scar-repair takes time!)

- ✓ It can be recognized as skin by its DNA and biology.
- ✓ There are 3 separate layers (containing different tissue) that function as one.

So all in all, your **skin is an extremely important organ** that deserves your conscious care.

<u>**Note:**</u>   1) Please understand that sun tanning and sun beds do not increase melanin in the skin. Tanning burns and damages your skin and can cause skin cancers.

2) Vitamin D is made when your brain detects sunlight through your pupils. Gaze (but don't stare) at the rising <u>sun in the dawn sky</u> for about 20 minutes without sunglasses. Your brain will pick up the cue to make vitamin D. In winter when the sky is clouded this process becomes more difficult and Seasonal Affective Disorder (SAD) can result. Sufferers get depressed, anxious, open to infection and even suicidal. (Vitamin D supplementation is definitely recommended in this case.)

Here's a fact that may interest you: elephant skin is very wrinkled…why? This is an evolutionary genetic adaptation to increase thickness and surface area and allow water to be trapped between the folds. It helps to regulate temperature and reduce dehydration in the animal's hot environment. Elephants don't have sweat glands like us… one of the reasons they love to spray water over themselves and bathe in cooling mud. ☺

> ➢ **My teenager has acne. What do you suggest?**

Teenagers have raging hormones. A cooling diet with plenty of water, fresh air and sleep will help a lot. First off, sit your teenager down and explain that topical products will only help short term ... if at all. That smoking (including passive smoking,) coffee, alcohol and 'recreational' drugs add to toxic overload and should be avoided. That what they eat becomes them and will inevitably appear on their faces! Their skins are working at top speed trying to remove excess hormones ... so for the best results they should do everything they can to support this effort.

Let's start with diet:

- ✓ Increase their vegetable and fresh fruit intake.
- ✓ Eliminate all sodas, 'energy' and other caffeinated drinks.
- ✓ Drink 100% fresh fruit juices in a 1/3 juice to 2/3 cold water ratio.
- ✓ Reduce fatty, refined and sugary choices ... burgers, hotdogs, corndogs, cakes, candy and cookies and replace with whole grain and home-made substitutes. Have them make lettuce wraps or help them make Thai veggie spring rolls. Ezekial bread and tortillas make awesome substitutes. Look for whole grain and 100% pasture-raised ground beef/bison and no-nitrite/nitrate options for burgers and wieners.
- ✓ Whole grain sandwiches with a few slices of a natural cheese (not Velveeta or over-processed varieties) and/or

organic peanut, cashew or almond butter make a great snack.

✓ Chicken and fish with 2 to 3 servings of different vegetables are a perfect dinner or lunch.

✓ Avoid go-to packaged Mac and cheese ... home-made with healthy ingredients and stuffed with one or two layers of veggies: chopped leafy greens, broccoli, carrots, mushrooms etc are tasty and add dense nutrition in the place of empty calories.

Keep skin clean:

✓ Use warm water and soap – *Zum Bars* or any other natural soap works well. Avoid harsh soap and so-called "cleansing" bars ... they will strip the natural acid mantle of the skin and make matters worse.

✓ Add a few drops of fresh-squeezed lemon or lime to cool water for rinsing. This is a perfect astringent.

✓ Rose water (found in most health stores and pharmacies) is an inexpensive and wonderful facial cleanser. Apply with cotton wool pads.

✓ Organic jojoba oil (find in health food stores ... buy the smallest bottle as it goes a long way) is a perfect moisturizer for skins of any age. Use clean fingertips to smooth a few drops at a time over the face and neck. Jojoba oil is the closest in chemical composition to our own sebum ... the oil produced by our skins ... and will maintain the essential acid mantle.

✓ Remember that your skin is **not an organ of digestion**! It is incapable of digesting heavy creams and butters for use by the deep layer skin cells. These products have largely false claims and tend to block pores and cause dirt build up.

✓ However, **your skin can and does absorb** what you place on it, so be very careful of what you choose. Read ingredient lists carefully. I recommend steering clear of any ingredients you wouldn't eat: preservatives you don't recognize as food and petro-chemical industry ingredients such as mineral oil (in many baby and facial products,) and petroleum jelly (lip-ice and many balms.) Try making balms and skincare oils yourself ... a few drops of organic rosemary, lavender or tangerine essential oil (EO) in a small bottle of Jojoba oil is a blissful moisturizer on warm skin ... including your face.

✓ My Mum used to say she could see on a friend's face that her feet were aching! A hot basin of water with 2T of Epsom salts and 1T English mustard powder dissolved in the water, makes an awesome and relaxing foot soak for tired shoe-sore feet. A few drops of peppermint EO in Jojoba oil ... just mix directly in your palm ...rubbed onto warm dry legs and feet, is both soothing and invigorating. Guaranteed to reduce lines on your face as well! Do a side-by-side soak with your teen … and chat about the day together.

<u>Stay active</u>. Exercise …

- ✓ that induces sweating will help to clear out pores. Make sure to shower/bathe every day to support skin health.
- ✓ will help to use up stress hormones (cortisol) and clear them from the body.
- ✓ will support better sleep, which in turn supports more efficient detox of the skin and other organs.
- ✓ will help to keep blood sugar balanced and this will reduce the possibility of weight gain.

Chapter 6: Notes, Thoughts, Actions and Goals

<u>Answers to questions you wouldn't think to ask.</u>

Chapter 7

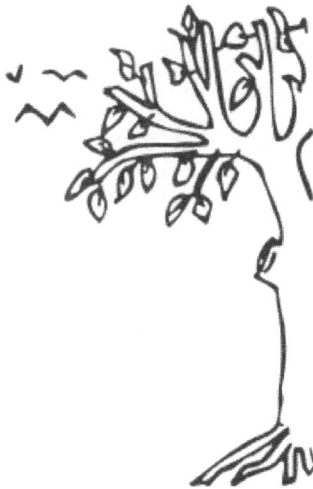

Miscellaneous Lifestyle Questions

> ➤ **How can I stay healthy when I travel?**

When we travel we experience more stress than usual. Have you ever become constipated when on holiday? This is because your digestive system slows down when you're stressed. There are a number of things you need to do to stay healthy and enjoy your trip, especially when flying.

1. **Food**
- ☝ My preference for any flight serving meals, is vegan, vegetarian, Thai or Asian … I avoid red meat and reduce the amount of bread/rolls, etc. I like to carry a few pieces of fresh fruit on board to eat … just be sure to eat it all or leave it on board. Most countries won't let you bring raw produce in through customs.
- ☝ On a long haul flight, avoid alcohol and coffee – both will dehydrate you, which means you won't sleep as well and will feel the effects of jetlag more.
- ☝ Juice Plus+® Chewables and Complete snack bars are my go-to for an in-between bite on overnight flights. They have high protein and fiber without high sugar, fat and carbs.

2. **Water**
- ☝ Keep hydrated … you need even more water than usual because of air-conditioning and especially airplane cabin dryness. I suggest bottled water in any foreign country.

You do not want a tummy bug spoiling your time away. Be careful of getting water in your mouth while showering or brushing your teeth … and watch out for ice cubes!

3. Routine and Sleep

- Try to get into the arrival time zone immediately you board the plane. Meaning if it is 11 pm at your destination when you board, go to sleep immediately. If you arrive at 3pm, go walking and do afternoon tourist or business things until it's time for dinner and then bed by 10pm.

- Add 5 drops of lavender EO to a 4 oz spritzer of spring water (airport security will confiscate anything larger!) It's wonderfully rehydrating and calming when spritzed directly onto your face (also for irritable children, your hubby, etc) before and during sleep on long flights or car trips. Breathe in deeply … you'll relax!

- I carry a small bottle of my favorite rosewater freshener, cotton wool pads and moisturizer in my overnight bag to clean my face before attempting to sleep on a plane. The routine of brushing my teeth and pampering my face focuses me on sleep.

- Carry a large t-shirt and non-binding pants to change into … I also like thick socks … an eye-cover mask and ear plugs or headphones. You're much more likely to drop off to sleep when your world is dark and quiet.

🖐 I discovered that putting an inflatable neck cushion on backwards (put it on so that the opening is behind your neck) works better to prevent my head lolling forward … that neck breaking jerk that only serves to wake you up again!

4. Exercise

🖐 On long flights be sure to do the exercises in the in-flight magazine. Ankle and knee flexing, ankle circles, knee lifts while seated … all are necessary to relieve possible thromboses. Having your knees, ankles and hips bent for long periods at a time stops blood flow and can be dangerous.

🖐 If you wake, get up, walk about the plane and do some yoga stretches if possible. I often have a group of passengers joining me with breathing and stretching at the back of the plane! It's fun … you meet nice people.

🖐 At your destination, try to get some walking in before you hit the sack each night. It will help you overcome jetlag faster and keep you from gaining vacation weight.

5. Health Aids

🖐 *"Thieves"* the Young Living EO blend is great to breathe in during a long flight or car ride. It keeps the nasal passages open and will guard against cold and flu viruses in your new environment.

- ❧ I recommend chelated Magnesium citrate tablets (no M. oxide, M. stearate or fillers ... *Albio*n makes well-formulated products) both as a muscle relaxant for "restless leg syndrome" and to support regularity and/or the 3-herbal blend - *"Triphala"* for colon toning and regularity. Neither is an aperient nor laxative, so you will not go from constipation to diarrhea and back again.

- ❧ A new environment, people around you with coughs and your stressed immune system, equate to the possibility of catching a pesky cold! A great cold/flu remedy is *"Oscillococcinum"* ... a homeopathic available from health stores, Walmart, and more. Take as recommended, at the first sign of a scratchy throat or wet sneeze. I also carry *"Echinaforce"* herbal drops for colds or flu... and plenty of tissues and *"Ricola"* natural herb lozenges ... great for easing a dry throat and mouth while traveling.

- ❧ Eat as closely as you can to your usual fare, but don't let that stop you sampling foreign delicacies.

- ❧ Take your trusty Juice Plus+® consistently ... it will keep supporting your immune system while you're traveling anywhere in the world.

CHOOSE TO BE HEALTHY

> ## Do my genes decide my health?

Up until the turn of this last century, we thought they did. The good news is that with the unraveling of the genetic code another field of study ... Epigenetics or Epigenomics ... was born. We now know that we can switch good genes on and bad genes off by making the kind of lifestyle changes espoused in this book.

Nutrition is of special significance in this regard. When we flood our systems day in and day out with dense, whole plant-based nutrition, we can reduce the everyday ravages of oxidative stress. Without constant anti-oxidant support free radicals cause untold damage to cells.

Here's an analogy: A free radical throws a fire bomb at your house. It may hit the outside wall and begin burning there. The fire department may be able to put this and similar fires out. However, when the fire bomb goes through a window and begins burning inside, the people in your home ... the DNA of your family ... may be burnt or damaged.

The fire department is your immune system ... working flat out for you day and night for your entire life. If your environment, your food choices, your lack of water and sleep and high stress job create too many free radicals ... they will overwhelm your immune system, and your health will begin to fail.

Using the guidance of this book will literally help you take back your health, keep your immune system fighting fit and reduce potential damage to your precious cells and your genes. If genes are damaged or if they're healthy, they decide your destiny. It's your choice: keep them safe ... the good turned on and the bad turned off and you stand a much better chance of living a long healthy life.

> ➤ **What causes Osteoporosis?**

Osteoporosis and its precursor osteopenia is a loss of bone density and mineralization resulting in thinning of the bones. I remember my nursing sister mother telling me a patient of hers had broken her hip. What was odd at the time, was she said that she wasn't sure if the woman had fallen first or whether her hip had given in first, causing a fall. Later when I learned about osteoporosis, I recalled this conversation. Which comes first: the fall or the fracture? Hip fractures and aging seem to go together these days ... but they needn't!

Let's look at the biology behind bone density.

Our cells are at their **healthiest when** they are at a pH of around 7.30 to 7.45, in other words, **very slightly alkaline**. If we eat sugary, fatty and meat-laden diets (think fatty ACIDS and amino ACIDS) we can shift this delicate balance towards a more acidic cell environment. I call this *Acidosis*.

Sodas are particularly dangerous because of their ingredients … lots of added sugar, often high fructose corn syrup, acidic preservatives such as citric and phosphoric acid, sodium benzoate, often caffeine and chemical flavors and colors. They **contain no nutrients** at all, but **are laden with potential toxins** … very good reason to eliminate them from your and your kids' diets. Drink water instead.

A pediatrician colleague told me recently that many children she sees nowadays in her practice, have clean-break fractures, instead of the "green-stick" fractures she used to see years ago, where the bones bent slightly, but did not break. She believes it is yet another symptom of the nutrient-deprived, sugar-laden and refined diets of our kids.

When *Acidosis* occurs, Mother Nature, liking balance, will shift the body back towards alkalinity, by **transferring minerals from the bones** where they belong. Over time, this constant rebalancing to keep us healthy causes our bones to demineralize and get thin and brittle … first osteopenia and later full-blown osteoporosis. It appears to be a condition of the aged, but it takes a long time to develop. Thus seniors are more at risk for bone fractures when they fall, or for falling because of collapsing bones (as in my Mom's story.) Worse, all too often, a fractured hip caused by osteoporosis, results in death.

When we **eat a plant-based diet**, we keep our **bodies more alkaline and therefore healthier**. It's as easy as that! There are naturally more minerals (calcium, potassium, magnesium and so on) in plants than in dairy. Most milk is fortified with calcium as the cows are not pasture-fed. Once I shifted from an acidic high-dairy diet to a conscious and healthy plant-based diet, I reversed my own bone density scores. Once we support our bodies, they can heal us.

The second component of bone loss, after good nutrition, is a **lack of weight-bearing exercise**. As we bear weight, our muscles pull against our bones and the bones pull back. As we have seen before, when our bodies are in need of help AND THEY ARE SUPPORTED, they will heal or build themselves in answer to our needs. Stronger muscles lead to stronger bones. Yoga, swimming, walking, gardening, jogging, dancing and rowing are wonderful bone strengthening and muscle toning exercises for seniors in need of upping bone density scores.

Think of the large herbivores of this world ... horses, elephants, rhinos, hippos, even whales ... not only are they never obese, they also have strong and supple bones. Why? They eat plants, never stop exercising, drink plenty of water, roam in the sunshine and avoid our human stressors! Does that make you think? ☺

> ➤ **Why is gut health so important?**

Any symptoms of gut ill-health … bloating, gas, constipation, diarrhea, pain, ulceration and so on are debilitating. From this point alone, gut health is important.

This set of symptoms, has now been termed *"Leaky Gut Syndrome."* Although it is not yet studied in medical schools, many gastroenterologists are recognizing a pattern … which is this: first these symptoms appear, after which they are sometimes followed by an auto-immune disease such as Multiple Sclerosis, Chronic Fatigue Syndrome, Rheumatoid Arthritis, Celiac Disease, Hashimoto's Thyroiditis and more.

It is thought that either:

the gut lining becomes permeable to undigested food molecules which cross directly into the bloodstream and are then attacked by our immune systems, or the undigested and decaying food particles release toxins that make the lining permeable. Either way, once pinprick holes appear in the colon walls, food molecules can move out freely into the blood.

Our immune systems see these molecules as enemy combatants to be attacked and destroyed. The only problem is, that our food becomes us! When immune system "soldiers" discover these same food molecules making up our muscles, joints, thyroids, villi, nervous system, organs, etc …. they attack them too! Rather like the blind watchdog that attacks its own owner!

It is believed in some quarters that all auto immune diseases follow the same path … Gut-destroying food and/or steroid/antibiotic overuse …leads to "Leaky gut syndrome" … leads to all-out immune response … leads to one or other auto immune disease.

It is noteworthy that about 70% of our immune system resides in the gut. The **microbiome … made up of trillions of complementary bacteria** (that is … they **work for** us, not against us) … helps us to maintain a healthy balance between good and bad bacteria. Plants feed and strengthen the microbiome; processed 'foods' weaken it. Gut 'dysbiosis' occurs when the bad bacteria overwhelm the good ones … **Candida overgrowth** is one such result. Yet another example of how we compromise our own immune function with poor food choices.

What to do?

Before I recommend any course of action, I'd like to challenge YOU to write down what you think (or know) I am going to say! By this stage of the book, I'm guessing (hoping) that you will already have the answers. Cover the next paragraph … or just close the book … make your list and then see how close you are!

- ASAP, move to a plant-based diet … especially high in green-leafy vegetables, fiber, dense nutrition and anti-oxidants, and low in natural sugars and sodium.

CHOOSE TO BE HEALTHY

- ☙ If diet allows, add wild-caught, cold-ocean fish … cod, salmon, halibut and sea bass … all have healthy fats and some have Omega 3.
- ☙ Pasture-raised and organic eggs will also add Omega 3
- ☙ Eat many small meals rather than 1 or 2 large meals a day … and chew your food really well.
- ☙ Eliminate wheat and gluten-grains.
- ☙ Eliminate caffeine, alcohol and smoking.
- ☙ Drink the right amount of filtered water for your weight (see page xxx)
- ☙ Eliminate added and refined sugars, syrups, sodas.
- ☙ Eliminate all dairy.
- ☙ Add pro-biotics
- ☙ Make sure you get at least 8 hours of sleep … plus cat naps when needed.
- ☙ Do yoga for stretching and strength; walk and do breathing exercises to calm the nervous system and reduce stress. Swimming is another great option.
- ☙ Think happy thoughts … visualize a healthy, pink, smiling gut. I had one client who painted a big smile on her tummy. She said it helped her remain smiling and positive!
- ☙ Try some of the supportive therapies mentioned under the next question
- ☙ Furthermore, I suggest adding Juice Plus+® Vegetable, Fruit and Berry capsules or Chewables as well as the plant-based Juice Plus+® Omega Blend.

CHOOSE TO BE HEALTHY

My rationale for this recommendation is the compelling Juice Plus+® research on reduction of at least three of the major symptoms of all auto immune disease, namely:

- ✖ **systemic inflammation**
- ✖ **high levels of homocysteine and**
- ✖ **high levels of free radical damage**

(Ref page 106 - Juice Plus+® research findings.)

> ➢ **What other therapies are worthwhile?**

Personally I have a **chiropractic** session about every 5 to 6 weeks. I was developing scoliosis at one time, (probably because of favoring my injured right knee) but after having repeated chiropractic sessions over the years, my spine is now straight and I'm in a much better place.

Every now and then I feel the need of a **colonic session** … especially if I have binged over some celebration or other! Nowadays, my high fiber, plant-based diet is sufficient to keep me regular and I do not take any medications. I recommend colonics whenever a client has been on repeated anti-biotic, steroidal or chemo/radiation doses or is chronically constipated.

I recommend a good **massage** therapist … and either deep tissue or **Cranio-sacral** sessions once a month or bi-monthly.

Massages are wonderful to promote lymphatic drainage and reduce the stress of our everyday lives.

I am a **Reiki** Master and practice **Reflexology** as well as **Raindrop Technique**, which is a therapy using a sequence of Young Living essential oils along the spine. These therapies are all energy balancing in their own right and have wonderful effects. A major benefit is that they can be used to complement medical treatments and pre- and post-surgery, because they are non-invasive.

Yoga and breathing exercises are a great way for us to massage and tone our own muscles and organs and reduce high blood pressure naturally. Effectively used by seniors to reduce pain, children for stress reduction and focus and during pregnancy, they help us with strength, stretching, balance, centering and pulmonary health and as such, yoga can be regarded as a therapy.

Acupressure, Acupuncture, Magnetic Resonancing, Herbal support, Iridology and **Homeopathy** all need a mention.

While there are many other health-supporting therapies practiced by practitioners, these are best known to me.

> ➢ **What should I be asking my Doctor?**

Your doctor is in your service ... your doctor puts his or her considerable educational skill and experience to work for you ... but **YOU are still the one who is responsible for your own health.**

- Be sure to ask exactly what medications and treatments are being prescribed and why.
- If you want to move towards a more natural and preventative approach, discuss with your doctor exactly what you are doing. Chances are they will applaud your decision and be happy to support you, especially if it entails better nutrition. Blood screening is one way your doc will be able to measure your progress as you change your diet and lifestyle.
- Preferably don't be buying every new flavor-of-the-month "cure" from the health store. Most of the supplements out there have never been studied on humans for their cellular effects. The massive supplement industry relies on haphazard word of mouth, rather than gold standard and reliable research. When your doctor tells you not to take any supplements ... it is these products s/he is talking about!

Remember that most doctors learn nothing about nutrition and lifestyle "therapies" during their training. (They'll be the first to admit this too!) I remember chatting with a doctor about what I could offer his patients ... I was amused to see *"Nutrition for Dummies"* on his bookshelf. Needless to say, he was embarrassed! (It only just dawned on me, that maybe many doctors actually believe that nutrition is of no more importance than this!)

> ➢ **What's the difference between Allopathic and Naturopathic approaches to health?**

The **Allopathic, or Medical approach** is all about <u>treating</u> the <u>symptoms</u> of disease ... and treating <u>each organ and system as a separate entity</u>. (For example: heart, kidney, lungs etc ... there's a specialist doctor for each.) In order to be treated, you have to be sick. Prevention in this approach is limited to testing for already-existing symptoms.

The **Naturopathic approach** is to regard the person as having an <u>integrated mind, body and spirit</u>. From this viewpoint, therapies are focused on the whole person, are primarily <u>stress-reducing</u> and are **Preventative** in nature... you are treated before you have any symptoms, so that symptoms do not ever manifest.

There is a Catch-22 inherent in the naturopathic approach: If you never get a chronic disease while practicing prevention ... how do you know whether you'd have got one if you hadn't practiced prevention? I don't know about you, but I for one will be more than happy if I practice prevention and never know whether there might have been a different outcome had I not!!

If you are already chronically ill, your body, specifically your immune system, will be supported and built to where it can function as it is meant to on your behalf. For instance nutrition and energy-work focus on building the health of every cell in the body. When you feel physically well, you are more likely to have balanced emotional wellbeing, as well as a healthy brain and nervous system.

My school motto was: *"Mens sana in corpore sano."* Which means *"A healthy mind in a healthy body."*

I guess the seeds of naturopathy were planted further back than I had realized!

> ➤ **What do you think about journaling?**

I enjoy journaling. It's difficult to make it a daily habit, but it's so worth it. As a child I kept a diary about daily events …which make for interesting 'historical' reading! When we're healthy, we forget what poor health feels like … when we're ill we forget what good health feels like. **Journaling is a great way to track these feelings and our daily reality**. Whenever I go back to past journals I'm amazed at my journey, at how far I've come and at how much I've learned and used new information to make constructive changes.

A young client once said to me: *"I didn't know how unhealthy I was until I started to feel healthy again!"*

When we're young we're gung-ho about our health. I have so often heard: *"I'm really healthy. I don't have to care about what I eat!"*

I promise you, there will come a time when you wish you could go back and change both that attitude and outcome. If you have a journal to go back to, you will be able to see where changes began and what you were doing to cause them.

I worked at a local "Curves" earlier in my health career. One of the things I remember from their intake interview was this: What was your weight on your wedding day? What is your weight now? Subtract the one from the other and divide by the number of years between. You will find that you probably have added 1½ to 2 lbs of weight each year following your wedding date. If you keep a journal which includes your annual weight, you'll have a better handle on first being conscious of weight gain and secondly doing something constructive about it.

Appendix C offers you a free template of a typical journal page. You are welcome to copy the blanks, file them and use them to help you get into the groove. Have fun, use color and drawings or sketches to really make your journal work for you.

CHOOSE TO BE HEALTHY

> ➢ **What can I do to support the environment?**

This is a question I wish more people would ask! In our own small ways we can all do so much to create a wave of change ... for instance:

- ☺ Start using reusable cloth bags for groceries.
- ☺ Ask for paper sacks rather than plastic bags if you have not brought your own bags. (In South Africa we were all irritated when stores began charging 10c for every plastic bag needed by a customer ... but nowadays there isn't one torn bag hanging from a fence or thorn tree across the country! No one wants to pay for bags and any found lying about now have value. Littering was literally cured overnight.)
- ☺ Many stores now have compostable cutlery, picnic plates and cups. Most cities and many towns have parks departments which practice composting, even if you don't. (Plastic in our environment is now so pervasive that even pristine beach sand made by the volcanic eruption of Mt Kilauea in 2018 has been found to contain 21 'bits' of micro-plastics per 50gm of sand! We and the animals cannot help but ingest plastic. We have no idea of the potential long term damage/injury to us and our environment.)
- ☺ Many towns have curbside recycling ... separate your plastics, glass, paper, card and aluminum as required.

CHOOSE TO BE HEALTHY

☺ If you are buying more whole foods and produce, chances are you'll be throwing away far less packaging … good for you!

☺ Change to non-toxic or low-impact dish-washer and laundry soaps … and eliminate harsh detergents and household cleaning materials.

☺ Attend meetings of your local chamber of commerce and/or city hall to find out what they are doing about recycling, water needs, air pollution, open-space and park areas and so on.

☺ If you have a garden, go organic ASAP. Start by eliminating ALL toxic pesticides, herbicides, fungicides. Ask gardening/lawn and tree- and pest-service personnel to work with you or seek out those who will.

☺ Once your garden is organic, seed a patch of butterfly-enticing plants and flowers … set out bird feeders and water for wild life. Plant a bunch of sunflowers … feed yourself and your neighborhood birds and wildlife in the fall. You'll create a paradise for yourself and return lost habitat to local birds and small animals.

☺ Start a neighborhood environmental challenge … be creative! Meet your neighbor parties are fun!

> ➤ **Why do you recommend Juice Plus+®?**

When I first heard about Juice Plus+® it made perfect sense to me. I already knew about oxidation and free radical damage, but I also knew that eating large amounts of fruit would add too much sugar to my diet, although fruit and berries are wonderful sources of the anti-oxidants we need for good health. Juice **Plus+® Capsules contain no sugar as it is removed in a proprietary process.** It was a 'no-brainer' way to gain thousands of anti-oxidants without paying the price of excess sugar.

As a Naturopath I am especially impressed that the Juice Plus+® Company has gone to the trouble of giving the nod to so many medical research institutions around the world, to **do gold standard, primary research studies on the effects of their product in humans.**

The term "Gold standard" means that research is:

- Done on the product itself
- In human trials
- Subjects are randomized to
- Studies that are double-blind and
- Placebo-controlled.
- All findings are published in peer-reviewed journals.
- In addition there is no animal testing.

CHOOSE TO BE HEALTHY

<u>Research findings from 39 studies to date</u>, are:

- **Juice Plus+® is bioavailable** (it gets into the blood stream and from there into the cells where it does its work.
- **It significantly raises anti-oxidant and nutrient levels in the blood** (combatting free radical damage.)
- **It improves postoperative outcomes after molar surgery**.
- **It improves periodontal health** (gum bleeding and pocket depth.)
- **It decreases homocysteine** (an amino acid that when raised, is linked to heart disease, stroke, auto immune diseases and Alzheimer's Disease.)
- **It helps to maintain normal healthy elasticity of arteries**.
- **It protects lipids from oxidative damage**.
- **It increases both the number and the activity of circulating immune cells**.
- **It reduces DNA damage and has been shown to benefit functioning of several key genes** (the study of Epigenomics shows that genes can be switched on and off … you want the good ones turned on and the dangerous ones turned off!)
- **It increases skin micro-circulation, density, hydration and thickness**. (There's a distinctly healthy glow about those who have taken Juice Plus+® for a few months!)

- **It decreases several key biomarkers of systemic inflammation** (a silent condition that is key to a number of health issues.)
- **Quality of life of ovarian cancer survivors improves**.
- **It improves the insulin resistance in overweight boys, reduces abdominal fat and increases lean muscle mass**.
- **It improves lung function** even in smokers.

These findings, together with my own health experience, have made a believer of me.

The *Shred-10 program* (mentioned in Chapter 4) is effective for reducing Metabolic Syndrome and teaching better eating and lifestyle habits. Central to the program is Juice Plus+® Complete which adds a further 15 whole plants to the 30 provided by the Vegetable, Fruit and Berry capsule blends. I have personal experience of many of my clients gaining better control of their blood glucose after adding Complete and cleaning up their diets. The Nemours Children's health study showed the same result.

The Healthy Starts for Families program gives one child FREE product when one adult buys the product. Parents choose from either Capsules or Chewables for themselves and their children. I love being able to offer this program. It means that a family of four can gain the benefit of Juice Plus+® for the price of two. Children aged 4 to 18 may remain on the program for 4 years, which gives them all the benefits mentioned above. This is key to their foundational good health.

CHOOSE TO BE HEALTHY

The Juice Plus+® Company develops many tools for its Partners (Independent franchise owners), among which is:

"One Simple Change" … a short and simple program that when followed, will result in beneficial lifestyle changes.

1. Eat a plant-based and whole food diet.
2. Get 8 hours of sleep a night.
3. Drink water as recommended
4. Exercise every day.
5. Have some quiet, introspective time every day (**See Appendix D for a 7-Day abundance affirmation exercise**.)

This is a company and product range that I trust … both with my own and my clients' health. In fact I've heard many a doctor say that he feels it would be unethical NOT to tell his patients about Juice Plus+® when it has so much to recommend it.

Armed with the knowledge in this book, you are now in a great position to actively **Choose Health and Make it your #1 priority**.

Best wishes with your journey.

Chapter 7: Notes, Thoughts, Actions and Goals

CHOOSE TO BE HEALTHY

<u>60 + USEFUL HEALTH TIPS AND HINTS</u>

Chapter 8

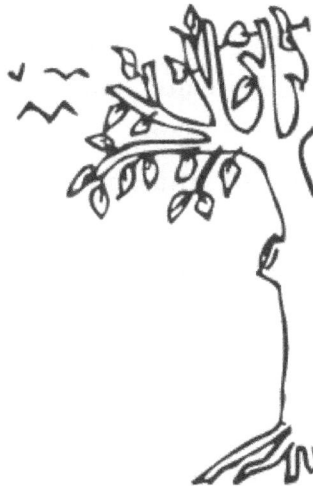

60 + USEFUL HEALTH TIPS AND HINTS

Healthy Eating:

1. *"Eat to live not live to eat."* (Socrates 400 BC)

2. If you want to endear yourself to your family, look for raw vegan dessert recipes online. These add whole food, are plant-based and scrumptious alternatives to sugary, cooked pies and so on. Pie bases can be made with almond or hazelnut meal and Juice Plus+® Complete powder and mashed dates as the sweet binding agent. Check out this website **www.onegreenplanet.org** … there are also many others.

3. *"The food that you eat can either be the safest and most powerful form of medicine or the slowest form of poison"* (Ann Wigmore – Holistic health practitioner and raw food advocate.)

4. Squeeze excess citrus fruit and freeze 1T per cube in freezer ice trays. Use a lemon 'ice-block' in water, or when cooking fish, chicken, pasta sauces and so on.

5. *"Eat whole food, not too much, mainly plants."* (Michael Pollan)

6. Bridge your everyday nutrition gaps with Juice Plus+®.

7. Ask your local grocer to stock specific healthy options/products for you. Then make sure you buy them from the grocer so that they will continue stocking that item. With all the competition out there, grocers will be happy to help.

8. Consider joining a local organic produce co-op. Look in *Meetup* for groups, search at local farmer's markets and your town Chamber of Commerce. At least buy local and in season whenever possible. Start your own co-op, or healthy eating Meetup and meet new like-minded people in your area.

9. **Don't ever reward yourself with food**. Buy something small but meaningful … or take a friend out to a movie, show, dancing … have fun. Food "rewards" are not likely to be healthy!

   So saying, have a little portion of cake or dessert or chocolate when you feel like it … don't deprive yourself to the extent that you start cravings. **Eat healthy 98% of the time!**

10. Check old favorite recipes for poor nutrition choices.

✓ Most desserts taste even better with half the sugar…add some ground spice for flavor.

✓ Replace margarine and lard with a little coconut or olive oil.

✓ Bake with more whole-grain flours than refined and bleached white flour.

✓ If using gluten-free meals/flours, try ***"Pamela's No-Gum Baking Binder"*** at a ratio of 1t per cup of flour. Xanthum gum is another option, but I prefer the texture of muffins, cookies, breads and cake using the "No-Gum" alternative.

11. Replace artificial colorants and flavorings with spices or berries wherever possible (eg. blueberries and cranberries in muffins, fresh mango or beet juice for a pink color, beets in brownies, turmeric for yellow rice.)

12. Experiment with grated zucchini, carrots, beets and greens in pasta sauces, pureed fresh pineapple, mango, pear and apple or whole fresh berries in cookies, cakes, muffins and breads. Try to substitute wet ingredients for wet in the original recipe. This is the perfect way to add sweetness and texture, while at the same time adding fiber, anti-oxidants and a range of vitamins and minerals … naturally. Google a veggie in a recipe (eg recipe for cake using carrots or beets?)

13. If you have a pressure cooker, cook up batches of dried chick peas, beans and lentils for freezing and later use. In the pressure cooker, soak a sack of your choice of bean, covered in water, overnight. Check after an hour or so – add more water if needed. Pour off the soaking water and re-cover with filtered water. Do not add salt or seasoning. Close the pressure cooker lid and bring contents to the boil. You will see the pressure gauge start to sputter. Immediately switch off the plate and remove the cooker. Leave it to cool completely before opening. The beans will be done perfectly with minimal electricity use. I bag and freeze cooked beans in gallon or quart-sized Ziplock bags … for use as hummus, in soups, salads, bakes, for Mexican sides, for beans and rice. I

season appropriately only when I use the beans, because cooking will draw seasoning – especially salt – into the bean and you'll need more later when you eat them. My seasonings of choice are ground cumin, onion and garlic powder, fresh garlic, lemon and lime juice, cracked coriander, cilantro, parsley, tomato salsa or spaghetti sauce, chili powder or flakes, black pepper and finally salt to taste.

Healthy Rehydrating

14. **Use water to rehydrate** … not sodas, not coffee, not alcohol … divide your real body weight by 2 … this is the amount in ounces you need for wonderful, energetic health every day. Water is a part of almost every process in our bodies. When we don't drink enough, water is reabsorbed from our colons … making us constipated … and from other areas … creating brain fog, kidney issues, wrinkled skin and so on. Athletes need even more!

15. To encourage more water drinking, place edible flowers or single berries into the cubes of an ice tray, fill with Club soda or Perrier water and freeze. Use whenever ice is needed.

CHOOSE TO BE HEALTHY

Healthy Shopping

16. Read <u>ingredient labels</u> as though your life depended on it… because it does! Nutrition labels are not as important.

17. When reading ingredient lists, "-<u>ose</u>" indicates a sugar (malt<u>ose</u> sucr<u>ose</u>, fruct<u>ose</u> and so on.) Manufacturers know we are being warned against excess sugar, so they rename products to disguise them. They also add sugar in syrup form. Be a wise and wiley coyote!

18. When you see *gluten-free, sugar-free* or *fat-free* on packaging, check the ingredient list carefully. Manufacturers will substitute all sorts of chemical additives to recreate the taste and mouth feel of the removed ingredient. Fat-free yoghurt for instance quite often has twice the amount of sugar as original yoghurts. Sugar-free almost always means added artificial sweeteners which are toxic to our brains (eg. Acelsulfame, sucralose, Splenda, aspartame.)

19. Don't believe in the saying: "Everything in moderation." Cocaine, heroin and sugar have the same influence on the brain! All three cause addiction and damage. You probably don't go near the first two … **please stay away from added refined sugar as well**. Manufacturers add untold amounts and varieties to babies' and children's food products. If you're a cynic, you might think they want to addict our kiddos to their products! Mmmm?

20. I buy large containers of ground onion, garlic and cumin powder (I use these as a base in almost all savory dishes.) I buy all other spices or seeds in small containers because the fresher your spices are the healthier and tastier your finished dishes.

21. Buy kale 1 or 2 bunches at a time or spinach/kale in bags/boxes. It is a really versatile and healthy addition to many savory recipes. Slice it up and add it to sauces for pasta, as narrow layers in bakes and macaroni cheese; sauté and add to fresh ground meat for burgers and to soups or egg dishes. It's tasty raw in salads too. Check out the recipes in Chapter 9.

22. Turn whole flour into self-raising flour by adding 1t of baking powder for every 1C of flour in your recipe. Look for aluminum-free baking powder … it's readily available at grocers.

23. Stevia is a good non-calorific sweetener to substitute for refined sugar. It is an herb, is not artificial and is 200 times sweeter than sugar, so a little goes a long way. ("Truvia" however, is an artificial creation made of erythritol, flavoring and stevia. Preferably avoid it!) Unless children are obese, let them have organic honey, molasses, maple syrup and organic brown sugar rather than stevia. But remember that all added sugar is still empty calories, no matter how organic and whole!

Healthy Lifestyle

24. *"When your blood sugar is balanced, you have will power."* (Dr Mitra Ray)

    Meaning: You don't feel hungry when your blood sugar is balanced. When your food contains fiber, protein and little to no added sugar, your blood glucose rises slowly and your pancreas secretes just enough insulin to deal with the small amount of ingested sugar. This food also takes longer to digest, so there are no spikes of hunger, followed by a crash. When you eat that sugary donut for breakfast, your blood glucose spikes and you will soon crash and then feel desperately hungry again.

    This is because as soon as your pancreas detects sugar bounding about in your blood stream, it secretes insulin to get the sugar out of your blood. **Sugar is toxic to your kidneys**. Once the sugar is gone, your brain shouts for more and the cycle begins again. So ... have meals and snacks that contain lots of fiber and dense nutrition so you don't feel hungry. **Avoid sugary options that spike your blood glucose and destroy your *will power***. Eat a piece of fruit or drink a glass of water before going to buy food.

25. Don't skip breakfast ... you don't need to eat much, but make sure you choose to eat nutrient-dense food. Without a healthy breakfast you are more likely to grab empty calories by mid-morning, because you are

ravenous and your brain is screaming for fuel! I have included some great breakfast recipes (in Chapter 9) that you can make ahead and keep stored. Cooked oatmeal, eggs and a bunch of braised veggies are also good options. Some mornings I can't face an early breakfast … I drink a glass of warm water and lemon instead, and have a breakfast smoothie at 9.30 or 10am. Then generally lunch is mid-afternoon if at all and dinner around 5pm. **Don't eat if you're not hungry.**

26. If you're **feeling hungry, first drink a glass of water** … you **may be mistaking the cue for thirst**. You are far more likely to be in need of water than food!

27. **Eat slowly and chew really well** on small bites of food. That way you start digestion in your mouth and probably won't ever have heartburn or acid reflux … especially if you are careful of your food combinations. (See **Appendix B** for a chart on optimal combinations.) You will also feel full faster … a great aid if you want to lose weight. Remember that your stomach is only about as big as your fist. And a child's fist is even smaller!

28. **Your senses are a part of your digestive system!** When you prepare your own food from scratch, you see it, you hear it being cut, you smell it … as a chef you also taste often. All these senses help your body to prepare for the coming food. I find I eat far less when I prepare my own food … I fill up on the glorious aromas!

29. For **a quick heartburn or acid reflux fix** that won't change your stomach juice chemistry … eat a stick of raw celery. Sleeping with your head slightly raised while lying on your left side also helps. Avoid antacids … they neutralize necessary gastric juice making digestion less efficient.

Healthy Systems

30. *"When the heart is at ease, the body is healthy."* (Chinese proverb.) Your amazing fist-sized heart pumps at a rate of 100,000 times a day, moving about 2,000 gals of blood through 60,000 miles of blood vessels every day! Practice the steps to health ("one Simple Change") at the end of Chapter 7 to keep your cardio-vascular system and your incredible athletic heart … as healthy as you can.

31. For better brain health, regard your brain as a muscle that needs and enjoys exercise and variety. Choose a new route home as often as you can; learn a new language; dance at home or take some lessons; actively search out new people to be around; have fun; take cooking or music lessons; read new authors; learn new skills. Eat clean, whole, plant-based and as healthy as possible. Drink plenty of filtered water. Exercise, have quiet, contemplative times and get all your sleep.

32. Alzheimer's Disease is also known as Type III Diabetes. Although we still do not know the cause of this dread disease, eliminating added sugar and eating a healthy

plant-based diet reduces Metabolic Syndrome (which is the precursor to Type II Diabetes.) What works for Type II, may well save you from Type III as well.

33. Your Immune System is designed to keep microbes out, kill mutated cells like those that initiate cancer, handle allergens, fight viruses and bacteria ... every second of every day that you live! Did you know that 10 teaspoons of sugar reduces your immune function by 50% and that 5 hours later your immune function has still not recovered. That's **18,000 seconds during which there's no watchdog at your door!** Very good reason to reduce added sugar and to watch sugar consumption.

34. The number of dialysis units that have sprung up is in direct proportion to the number of new diabetes sufferers. Again, sugar is the culprit. A healthy diet and lifestyle as laid out in this book will help to reverse Metabolic Syndrome (the precursor to Type II and gestational diabetes) as well as support better kidney health in current Diabetes sufferers.

Healthy Children

35. An egg a day works well to dispel depression and anxiety in children. The Sulphur and choline help support brain health.

36. *"Raise a grazer."* (Dr. Bill Sears) Let children nibble on healthy snacks whenever they're hungry. (See the *muffin pan* idea in Chapter 1.) Snacking a bit, then playing in

between, will naturally burn up calories. Your kiddos will be less likely to eat large meals that they cannot digest and you will set them up for healthy *metabolic reprogramming* ... which will change their tastes and set them up with health for life!

37. *"A few germs never hurt anyone."* (Germophobia) If we'd kept this in mind maybe anti-biotic resistance would not be such an issue today. A healthy lifestyle and eating habits in turn support a functioning immune system. Preferably don't use anti-biotic wipes on kids ... let their Immune systems learn to flex their muscles.

Exercise and Health

38. *"You cannot out-exercise a poor diet."*
Meaning: exercise and a poor diet will not support your efforts. You will get injured, sick and not recover effectively. To support exercise, you need a diet which provides fuel for performance AND for recovery.

39. *"Exercise should be regarded as a tribute to the heart."* (Gene Tunney – Professional boxer)

40. If you're injured, continue to exercise those limbs that can still be exercised. Breathing is an exercise when done consciously. Even if you have cancer, only a few of your trillion cells are likely to be involved ... tell your body that you still need it to work and support you, by exercising the rest of your trillion cells.

41. Buddy up if you're starting out with exercise. Do exercise during your work breaks ... up and down stairs; a little stretching; run out to your car and back a few times. Malls are great places to do laps! Not having a gym membership is no excuse! :-)

42. **Don't exercise on a full stomach.** Remember that your body handles one major function at a time. Digestion and physical activity don't go well together.

Healthy Sleep

43. **Sleep is too important to let negative thoughts interrupt and destroy it.** Every night before falling asleep, think of anything negative that happened during your day. Imagine sweeping it aside with your hand. Tell it: "Thanks for coming along to teach me xxx lesson ... now you have served your purpose and I no longer need you."
If it's something you need to talk over with someone to clear the air, ask: "Please give me guidance on how to discuss this with xxx, in a way that helps us both." Then let it go and relax and breathe as in Tip 45 on the next page. The universe will give you the answer in good time.

44. Another great just-before-sleep practice is to **list 10 people or things you are grateful for** ... or 5 to 10 things you loved about your day. Go to sleep with a smile and a

few deep breaths. (See **Appendix D for a 7-Day abundance affirmation exercise.**)

45. Do the following breathing exercise just before going to sleep … as well as any time you feel stressed (for instance before a speaking opp, or asking your boss for a raise.) It will serve to lower blood pressure, dissipate cortisol and adrenaline and help to clear your mind of unwanted thoughts.

    **Breathe in deeply and slowly through your nose counting in your mind 1,2,3,4,5,6,7 … hold for 1,2,3 … breathe out through your mouth, counting 1,2,3,4,5,6,7 … hold 1,2,3 before breathing in again and repeating for 5 more breaths.

Healthy Animals

46. Puppies love to chew … so to focus them away from precious shoes, table legs and so on, give them whole carrots and celery sticks to gnaw on. These are healthier and great to soothe itchy and painful gums during teething. For that matter babies do just as well with baby carrots and pieces of apple to mouth on.

47. Please **don't feed your animals with table scraps**, unless they are fresh, raw vegetables. I have a Veterinarian friend who showed me an x-ray of undigested cooked bones in the colon of a dog. The well-meaning owner was horrified (probably by the cost of the surgery as well as the pain the dog had to endure.)

48. **Cats are carnivores and need fresh and raw fish, meat and animal fat to thrive.** Do not feed them pasteurized milk. Only raw milk is okay – it still has natural digestive enzymes. (Google *Pottenger's Cat Study* to see the devastating effect of heat-processed food on cats.)

49. **Dogs are more omnivorous, but even so, they do not thrive on cooked food.** We feed ours 1T (Welsh Corgi) and 3T (German shepherd) ground turkey, grain-free pellets (*Blue, Nutrish, Beyond, Science Diet,* etc,) fresh and raw blended veggies every day and a raw egg every two weeks. Oh, and of course I give them a Juice Plus+® veggie and fruit capsule in their food as well. Our dogs are in great health, with sleek shiny coats, not over-weight, very energetic and never get sick.

50. When you choose a dog to be your companion, research the breed well before you buy or rescue. For instance an energetic Border Collie will be critically unhappy living in an apartment. **Match your lifestyle to your dog for the health and happiness of both of you** … and be prepared to exercise and feed your dog optimally for its breed.

Healthy Environment

51. For great and effective home-cleaning products … add 5 drops of any 3: pine, peppermint, eucalyptus, rosemary, oregano or lavender EOs to a spritzer bottle of water. Spritz counter tops, basins, toilets, baths, etc … including

floors and use paper towels or dedicated cloths to wipe down surfaces. It also smells great when used to clean inside your car, clothing or shoe cupboard. EO's perfumes are awesome and clean and they are natural anti-microbials that even crawling babies or animals can touch without harm.

52. Put a teaspoon of rosemary, eucalyptus or lavender EO into your washer instead of fabric softener for a gorgeous naturally perfumed result.

53. **A teaspoon of sugar** helps to keep cut flowers alive and pretty. When you first buy (or receive) them, use scissors to cut off about an inch of each stem under water … air bubbles get trapped in the stems and stop the flower sucking up water, so they fade sooner. Add the sugar to clean water … or change water weekly, adding sugar each time.

54. If you have naturally blonde hair, chamomile tea with a squeeze of lemon juice is a great hair rinse, while a rinse made with a black teabag is great on brown hair.

55. It's easy to grow a pot of herbs on a sunny windowsill. Choose from basil, parsley, rosemary, thyme, mint, oregano, cilantro and chives. Fresh herbs in our cooked and raw creations are so much tastier than dried. Tower Gardens by Juice Plus+® make gardening fun and foolproof. Read about and order yours from **www.taylers.juiceplus.com** … click the Tower Garden tab.

56. A quick **DIY for (toenail) fungus**, that is as effective as any OTC remedy, is the following: 1) Add equal parts <u>organic apple cider vinegar</u> and warm water to a bowl. 2) Soak infected nails for 30 minutes a day. 3) Remove toes/fingers and dry thoroughly with paper towels. 4) Repeat the process daily for 3 – 4 weeks for complete relief.

57. **Surround yourself with positive constructive people.** This is a surefire way to create harmony and joy in your life.

58. *"A good laugh and a long sleep are the best of possible cures for all ills."* (Irish proverb.) Laughter gives you a cardio workout; it dulls pain and reduces stress hormones like cortisol; it increases endorphins and happy hormones; it even increases anti-body producing cells and makes T-cells more effective! So find reason to belly laugh often. My Dad always maintained if I could laugh at myself, I'd never stop laughing. He's right … I'm a hoot!

59. This is specifically for all those care-givers who neglect themselves in favor of those they care for … as they tell us on an aircraft … put your own oxygen mask on first, then help the person next to you! Choose and then maintain good health … if for no better reason than YOU are worth it, and you won't be any use as a care-giver if you're sick too! *"Before healing others, heal yourself."* (Gambian saying.)

60. An opportunity only knocks once. The fact that you are reading this book/tip is an opportunity for you to ACT in your own interest. What will YOU do to make a positive change to your lifestyle from today on? ☺

61. *"Let food be they medicine and medicine be thy food."* (Unknown ... Attributed incorrectly to Hippocrates!

62. P.T. Barnum, the famous circus entrepreneur and philanthropist once said: *"The foundation of success in life is good health ... it is also the basis of happiness. A person cannot accumulate a fortune very well when he is sick!"* Enough said!

63. The last word goes to Will Rogers who said: ***"Even if you're on the right track, you'll get run over if you just sit there!"***

Chapter 8: Notes, Thoughts, Actions and Goals

CHOOSE TO BE HEALTHY

<u>Recipes</u>

Chapter 9

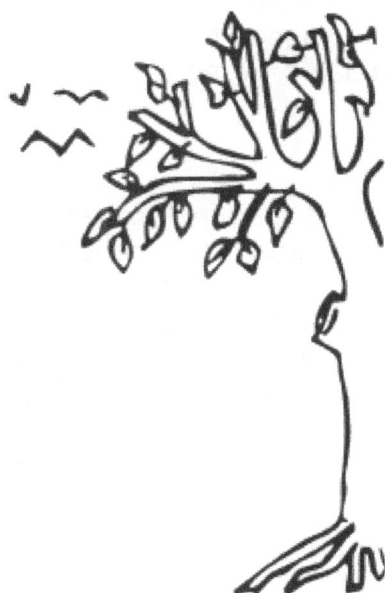

Recipes

These are a few of my go-to recipes specifically designed to add more whole plants to your daily diet. Play around with them to make them your own.
Above all …. Enjoy!

Breakfast

Bircher-Benner Muesli (Created in 1900's in a Swiss spa) (serves 3 to 4)

Mix together:
1C Muesli (see next recipe).
1 grated red apple (wash well but don't peel)
1C plain whole Greek yoghurt (can exchange for ½ C plant milk)
4 of each: Chopped dates, organic dried apricots /figs
½ t ground cinnamon
¼ t ground clove

Mix should be loose and spoonable … add fruit juice or more yoghurt/plant milk to desired taste and texture.
Soak overnight in fridge, in a sealed container.
Serve with plant milk and/or yoghurt for desired consistency.
Add fresh berries or sliced fresh fruit (banana, mango, grapes, papaya, pear) A drizzle of honey or organic maple syrup is nice.

Muesli

Set oven to 350 F or low broil.
On a baking tray spread a mix of:
3C organic uncooked rolled oats
½ C sliced almonds
½ C sesame seeds
1C walnut and pecan pieces (peanuts too if you like)
½ to 1C organic unsweetened shredded coconut

Place pan in middle of oven and stir muesli mix with a metal
egg-lift or long-handled spoon while it toasts … watch very
carefully … the natural fats brown and burn fast (especially if
you use the broil setting.)
When just turning golden brown (5 mins on broil and about 10
mins at 350 F) remove from oven and add:

1C raisins and/or sultanas (golden raisins)
½ C dried cranberries or cherries
½ C wheat germ flakes (if not gluten-sensitive)
½ C flax seeds

When fully cooled, store in an airtight canning jar or plastic
container in the fridge. Your muesli can also be put in Ziplock
plastic bags and stored in the freezer until ready to eat.

- A serving size is ½ C … add yoghurt, plant milk, fresh
  berries, honey … your choice.
- Muesli makes a great topping with added butter or
  coconut oil for fruit/berry cobblers.
- It can be added as part of the flour component, to muffins
  breads and biscotti.

Granola

Set oven to 350F
2C organic uncooked rolled oats
½ C organic unsweetened coconut flakes
½ C chopped nuts (almonds, walnuts, pecans)
½ C flax seeds (and/or sesame, hemp, chia seeds)
½ C honey
¼ C organic olive oil
¼ t ground ginger or cinnamon

Line a baking tray with parchment
Mix all ingredients till well coated … tip onto pan and spread loosely.
Bake on middle shelf till golden … stir a few times to make sure it doesn't burn.

Cool on the baking tray. Store in an airtight canister.
Serve with plant milk, as a topping over fresh berries and fruit, or with yoghurt … even with ice cream.

Salads

Raw Kale Salad

Wash a bunch of any kale (Curly, Russian purple, Dragon-leaf)
Your choice to cut away the thick midrib, or just slice it up fine.
Slice the greens and place in a bowl. Pour over:
1T organic olive oil
1T organic tamari (a form of soy) or low-sodium soy sauce
1 t cumin powder
1 t onion powder
½ - 1 t garlic powder
Juice of ½ lemon or lime

With clean, damp hands, massage the dressing into the kale
until the leaves darken and become softer to the touch. Make
sure you incorporate all the dressing at the bottom of the bowl.
Before serving sprinkle over
1T toasted sesame seeds (you can toast raw seeds yourself
(see Toasting in Chapter 2) or buy toasted seeds.

Optional additions:
½ C black beans
½ C chick peas
1T toasted sunflower seeds
1T finely grated Parmesan cheese or nutritional yeast.

CHOOSE TO BE HEALTHY

Layered Salad

This salad looks great in a glass bowl that shows the colorful layers.
Starting at the bottom ... ½ inch thick layers:
*Fresh chopped spinach or baby greens
*Sliced red peppers
*Sliced celery
*Sliced cocktail tomatoes
*Sliced cucumber
*Grated carrot (mix with 1 T orange /Clementine juice)
*Frozen baby peas
*3/4 C *Helmann's* mayonnaise mixed with ¼ C plant milk ...
spoon over the frozen peas to cover salad completely.
Serve when peas are fully thawed ... about 1 hour.

Thai Cole Slaw

Finely slice and mix:
¼ red cabbage
¼ green cabbage
¼ Napa cabbage
2 green onions
Grate 1-2 large carrots and immediately add:
2T Clementine or orange juice and
1 t ground ginger
(The citrus juice will stop your grated carrot oxidizing and going brown.)

Mix all veggies together and pour over:
1 T reduced sodium soy sauce
1 T olive oil
1 T toasted sesame seeds or sunflower seeds
Mix well and chill before serving.

Snacks

Lettuce (or Ezekial Tortilla) Wraps

Set out 9 separate small bowls of the following:
- Cut a large <u>carrot</u> into 3 equal pieces, slice lengthwise and then into matchstick pieces.
- Slice <u>cucumber</u> on the diagonal
- Slice <u>celery</u> finely on the diagonal
- Slice <u>cocktail tomatoes</u> in half
- Roughly slice 6 to 8 stalks of <u>cilantro</u>
- Sliced <u>avocado</u>
- Raw <u>bean or vegetable sprouts</u>
- 1 C <u>chick peas, black or red beans</u> … or a mix of your choice … seasoned with ½ t each ground cumin, onion, garlic powder (chili powder?) and 1 t lime juice
- ½ C Helmann's <u>Mayonnaise</u> mixed with 1 T peanut or almond butter (or plain mayo with a little black pepper … to your taste)

Tear leaves off a Romaine lettuce and place on a plate in the center of the small bowls.

"Paint" some mayo on a lettuce leaf and place a little of your choice of the other ingredients onto the leaf.
Roll the sides of the leaf over, and enjoy!
Alternatively, use warmed Ezekial tortillas in place of lettuce.

Smoothies

1 scoop Juice Plus+® Complete vanilla or chocolate powder
1 C plant milk or water
Your choice of fruit: mango and pear; orange and apple; apple and cinnamon; strawberry and banana; blueberries and mint …
1 handful of ice
Blend together till smooth.

CHOOSE TO BE HEALTHY

Hummus

Blend together till smooth:
1 C or can of chick peas (or ½ C each chick peas/black beans)
5 to 8 stalks of cilantro
Juice of 1 lemon
2T olive oil
1t ground cumin
1T toasted sesame seeds or sunflower seeds
1/3 C pecans
Add a little water if too thick.

For a nice flavor and nutrient change, add one of the following:
Avocado, fresh red pepper, chili flakes, sun-dried tomato.

Serve with toast, as a dip, as an addition to lettuce wraps, with fresh vegetable sticks … be creative! Hummus is an awesome protein source.

Crudites (Cruh-dee-tays)

On a large platter place groups of sliced or whole, colored fresh and raw veggies and fruit. Choose from:
**Strawberries, blueberries, pineapple, grapes, apple, mango, kiwi, melon and more.

**Celery, carrots, Bell peppers, broccoli, cauliflower, cocktail tomatoes, snow or snap peas and more.

**Organic plain Greek yoghurt flavored with a little honey or maple syrup and vanilla is tasty as a fruit dip. (If you have Juice Plus+® Complete vanilla powder, add 1T plus 1T plant milk to the dip.)

**Ranch dressing, hummus, avocado dip and seasoned mayo can be used as delicious veggie dips.

No-Bake Vegan Poppers

Pour ½ C boiling water over 8 pitted fresh dates
When soft, pour off (and drink) the water and mash with a fork
Add the following to dates and mix till all ingredients are coated:
1 C coconut cream
1 C toasted rolled oats
1/3 C organic peanut or almond butter
1/3 C chopped pecans and/or walnuts (almonds are good too)
1 scoop either Juice Plus+® Complete vanilla or Juice Plus+®
Complete chocolate powder*
¼ C raisins, sultanas or cranberries
½ C seeds – choose from chia, flax, hemp, sesame and
sunflower seeds
1t ground cinnamon
¼ t ground nutmeg

½ C organic, flaked and unsweetened coconut (for rolling)

Put mix into fridge for half an hour to make easier to roll.
Prepare a baking tray with parchment paper.
Roll 1T of mix into a popper and roll in the coconut flakes.
Place on the parchment
Place tray in fridge, when poppers are cold, store in an airtight
container for later eating.

**Option: if you do not have Juice Plus+® Complete smoothie
powder you can add 1/3 C organic cocoa powder or extra oats.
Hint: Wet your fingers slightly when rolling …the mix will be
easier to work with.

CHOOSE TO BE HEALTHY

Vegan Trail Mix

Mix together your selection of, or all of the following:

1 C mixed unsalted nuts (almonds, cashews, pecans, peanuts, walnuts)
1 C raisins
1 C dried cranberries
1 C organic coconut flakes (not shredded … it's too fine)
1 C mixed chopped dried fruit (berries, organic apricots, mango, banana, apple, etc Check packages to make sure there is <u>no sulphur dioxide</u> in dried fruit … it's a questionable preservative)
1 Juice Plus+® Complete Tart Cherry bar chopped into small bites
1 Juice Plus+® Complete Chocolate Fig bar chopped into small bites.
(The last two ingredients are an awesome addition to your trail mix, but are optional.)

Great in small Ziplock bags for school lunches, before or after sport, before during and after hikes, when traveling and so on.

Lunch or Dinner

Bean and Vegetable Soup

(This soup may be used in a 3-day fast … refer Chapter 6
Just leave out the beans and olive oil for the fast)

You'll need a LARGE pot for this … I freeze for later use …
alternatively you can split the recipe in half. Simmer till done.

4 cans of different beans (if organic, use liquid. If not organic,
drain and rinse beans)
Roughly chop/slice into bite-sized chunks:
4 onions (2 red, 2 white/yellow)
4 carrots
4 stalks of celery
3 yams/sweet potatoes
½ red cabbage
4 zucchini
1 - 2 bunches of kale
1 bunch of parsley or cilantro (or ½ and ½)
Add 2-4 containers of vegetable stock … add enough water to
completely cover vegetables.
Add:
3 T olive oil
Juice of 1 lemon
2 T each onion and cumin powder
1 T garlic powder
2-3 t salt (Himalayan pink salt is nice … also *Herbamare* by
A.Vogel) Check before serving … you may want to add more
salt.

Serve with toast and a green salad.

Creamy (Curried) Cauliflower Soup

(If you're not partial to curry, leave out curry powder)

1T Coconut or Olive oil
1 whole leek cleaned, trimmed and thinly sliced
2 cloves garlic ...crushed or finely chopped
Saute leek and garlic in oil till translucent
Add:
3 C water or vegetable broth
½ cauliflower roughly chopped
1-inch peeled and chopped, fresh ginger
2 t curry powder
1½ t turmeric
½ t salt
1 can coconut milk (about 450 ml)
¼ t ground cumin
½ t ground black pepper

Do not allow to boil ...the coconut milk will separate.
When hot, transfer to a blender and blend till smooth.

To serve, top with finely chopped fresh cilantro or parsley

(Turmeric and by association curry powder, because it contains turmeric, is a well-known Ayurvedic anti-inflammatory remedy. For best results eat/take turmeric with a little coconut oil and black pepper or honey. I prefer it in cooked dishes ... it's tasty in "yellow" rice with raisins or sultanas (golden raisins) added. Just add 2 t turmeric and a little salt to cooked, hot brown or white rice.)

CHOOSE TO BE HEALTHY

Stuffed squash

Set oven at 375 F
Bake a whole winter squash in a baking pan lined with foil - for
45 mins to 1 hour until a skewer goes in easily. (Delicata,
Butternut, Turban, Acorn, Sweet Dumpling squash all work
well.)
Halve and scoop out seeds, stuff with the following mixture:
Warm leftover brown rice or quinoa and mix with your choice of
chopped cooked veggies, raisins, nuts and seeds.
1 T coconut oil
Fresh black pepper and your choice of other seasonings.

Stuffed Baked Pasta Shells

Boil as per instructions 2-5 large pasta shells per person.
Drain when still slightly uncooked.
Set oven at 350 F
Stuff shells with a mix of chopped cooked veggies – include
mushrooms; shredded chicken; shrimp pieces; nuts; cooked or
canned beans; cooked brown rice, quinoa or lentils … your
choice… about 1 T of mix to a pasta shell.

Place a 1 inch layer of raw shredded spinach and kale in a
casserole dish … drizzle with 1 T olive oil.
Bed the stuffed pasta shells closely together onto the greens.

Pour over your choice of organic pasta sauce … depending on
the number of pasta shells, you will need 1 – 2 bottles of
prepared sauce … just cover the shells – don't drown them!
OR … If you're feeling creative … make your own sauce by
blending a can of tomatoes, sautéed Bell pepper, onion and
garlic, olive oil and mushrooms; fresh basil, thyme or rosemary,
black pepper and a drop of red wine or vodka. Keep the mix a
bit chunky.

CHOOSE TO BE HEALTHY

Veggie Mac and Cheese

Choose 5 or 6 greens and veggies … slice and dice finely …
sauté with a little coconut oil until transparent or soft.
Make your favorite Mac and Cheese recipe (from scratch of
course!) adding 2 thin (or thick) layers of cooked veggies
between Mac layers. Bake, eat and enjoy as normal!

Vegan Pasta Sauce

Sauté sliced Bell pepper, red and white onion and garlic in
1 – 2T olive oil
When onions are translucent,
Add sliced mushrooms
Fresh basil, thyme, coriander, parsley and/or rosemary
Sliced zucchini
Sliced carrot
Sliced celery
Freshly ground black pepper
1 – 2T red wine or vodka
Blend and add to cooked vegetable mix:
1 can of organic roasted tomatoes

Change it up:
1. Add chili flakes and serve with penne (Arrabiata)
2. Add cream for vegetarian Alfredo … just before serving.
   Do not boil … the sauce will curdle.
3. Serve over ravioli or stuff cooked Manicotti tubes
4. Try quinoa, vegetable or brown rice pastas
5. Serve over baked, scooped-out spaghetti squash – 375 F
   for 1 hour
6. Cook lasagna sheets and layer with this sauce. Bake at
   350 F for 30 mins.

Chapter 9: Notes, Thoughts, Actions and Goals (When did you make a specific recipe? How did you like it? How will you experiment to change it to your own taste?)

CHOOSE TO BE HEALTHY

APPENDICES

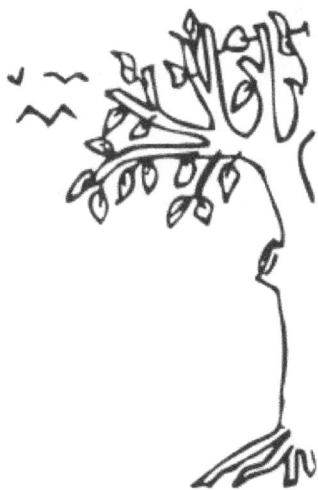

CHOOSE TO BE HEALTHY

Appendix A
WEEDING OUT THE SICKO'S

PHYTO's Fight for you (good choices)	SICKO's (poor choices)
Fresh and frozen fruit, veggies, berries	Hydrogenated and partially-hydrogenated oils & fats; trans fats
Fresh nuts and seeds	High fructose corn syrup (HFCS)
Organic first pressed olive oil, organic coconut oil, organic unsalted butter	Added sugars, (4g =1 packet) malt**ose**, fruct**ose**, lact**ose**, sucr**ose**, fruit syrups, galact**ose**, HFCS, corn syrup
Organic canned, unsweetened fruit, veggies and beans	Refined white flour (no fiber, low protein, no natural fat, high carb)
Dried pulses (lentils, beans, peas)	White rice (no fiber)
Organic juices (unsweetened) Mix 1/3 juice with 2/3 water	Artificial sweeteners (Aspartame, Equal, Nutrasweet, Sucralose, Acelsulfame)
Natural sweeteners – brown sugar, honey, agave, molasses, maple syrup Organic stevia – no-calorie, but natural.	Additives: colors (numbered eg Red #40); artificial flavors
Whole grains (3g or more fiber): millet, quinoa, amaranth, wheat and barley, oats, brown rice, spelt, buckwheat, rye	Preservatives such as Sodium Benzoate, BHT, Natamycin, Sulphur dioxide, EDTA
Wholegrain products (3g or more fiber): breads, pasta, muffins, waffles – but read ingredient lists for **Sicko** additives.	Fried foods: fat and carbs form hydro-carbons and acrylamide at high temp; also rancid, acidic and trans fats.
Organic pasture-raised poultry and eggs	Added sodium: S nitrate, S nitrite, MSG
Fresh and canned wild-caught salmon, tuna, sardines and other ocean fish.	Caffeine – in sodas, coffee, energy drinks and energy bars
Spring or filtered water –reverse osmosis	Fried, boiled and overcooked food
Plant milks: Organic and unsweetened - Westsoy (4g fiber), almond, coconut and rice milk	Highly processed plant oils: peanut, soy, canola, sunflower – calorie-dense, but nutrient-stripped.
Dairy products from 100% organic, pasture-raised animals (no antibiotics or growth hormones EVER.) milk, kefir, cream, butter, yoghurt, cheeses.	Dairy products from feed lot-raised cows: contain antibiotics, growth hormones, high gluten levels in feed create obesity and sickness: mastitis etc
Venison, bison, organic and pasture-raised lamb, beef. Too much IS NOT a good thing! Keep portion size to the palm of your hand, once or twice a week.	Red and "white" meat from feed lot-raised animals: see 'dairy products.' Animals are under constant stress and have high levels of cortisol & adrenaline. Acidic meat state can be measured.
Juice Plus+® nutraceutical products – contain whole, vine-ripened, sustainably and organically-grown produce.	Over-the-counter meds; unnecessary medication (side effects), artificial, isolated supplements (vitamins/minerals)

Appendix B

<u>FOOD COMBINING CHART</u> - especially helpful for anyone eating meat.

<u>Appendix C</u>: FOOD COMBINING GUIDELINES

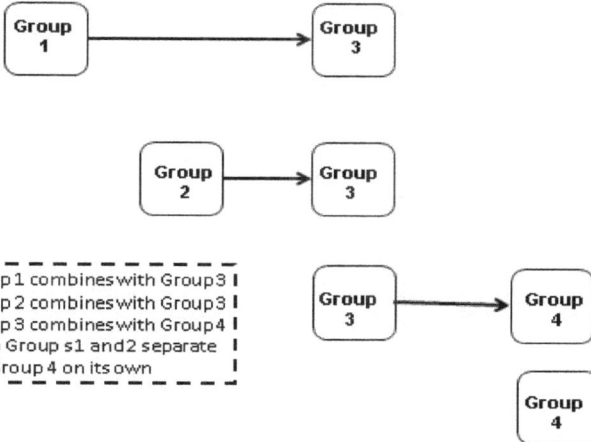

```
Group 1 combines with Group 3
Group 2 combines with Group 3
Group 3 combines with Group 4
Keep Group s1 and 2 separate
Eat Group 4 on its own
```

Group 1: All animal protein (red and white meats, fish, shellfish, dairy products)

Group 2: The 'whites': All carbohydrates and starches (potatoes, grains, dried beans, rice, pasta, flours, products made with grains and flours: breads, cookies, cakes; all sugars; milks made from grains: rice & soy)

Group 3: All colored vegetables (lettuces & leafy greens; root veggies: yams, carrots, sweet potatoes, beets, parsnips; cabbages, cauliflower, broccoli, tomatoes, bell peppers, winter and summer squashes, onion varieties, etc; all fresh and dried herbs & spices.

Group 4: All fruits and berries may be combined with Group 3; melons and cucumber are best eaten alone ... wait 20 minutes before eating any other food; preferably eat fruit and berries raw to maintain their alkalinity. Cooking plants from this group turns them acidic.

149

CHOOSE TO BE HEALTHY

Appendix C (You are welcome to make copies of this page for daily use.)

<u>**DAILY EATING AND LIFESTYLE JOURNAL**</u> (Draw, doodle, use color, have FUN!)

NAME: DAY & DATE:

BREAKFAST:

MORNING SNACK:

LUNCH:

AFTERNOON SNACK:

DINNER:

EXERCISE:

MEDICATIONS &/OR SUPPLEMENTS:

WATER CONSUMPTION:

STRESS-RELIEVING ACTIVITIES (Stretching, meditation, a bath, reading, etc):

PERSONAL NOTES (Current weight; Emotions, Physical well-being, Energy levels, Sleep patterns, Goals achieved? What can you Celebrate? What are you Grateful for? Is journaling easy or hard ... why? etc)

Appendix D

<u>7-Day Affirmation Exercise: Drawing Abundance</u>

The universe provides for all of us according to our needs. We are told in the Bible to "Ask and you shall receive." Why then do we so often feel guilt-stricken when asking for things for ourselves?

Try this 7-Day exercise on your own, or with a friend or two to expand your experience. Make sure you are not interrupted … this is your quiet time…it'll take you about 15 minutes.

♦ Choose the same time, every day for one week. Early morning, before starting your day, is perfect.
♦ Switch your cell off.
♦ Sit in a comfortable chair or lie in bed and relax, legs uncrossed and hands open on your thighs or at your sides.
♦ Breathe in deeply and smoothly through your nose counting in your mind 1,2,3,4,5,6,7 … hold for 1,2,3 … breathe out through your mouth, counting 1,2,3,4,5,6,7 … hold 1,2,3 before breathing in again and repeating for 5 more breaths.
♦ Say out loud, the affirmation for the day. Repeat the affirmation out loud, 3 times, then close your eyes and repeat it 3 times, slowly in your mind, while continuing to breathe.
♦ Remain quiet and relaxed, breathing slowly and deeply for another 5 breaths.
♦ On each day after completing the above steps, write down what you are focusing on for that day, for example, on Day 1 … list at least 20 of your blessings and think about how thy bless your life (Garth, my beloved dogs, my family, my friends …); on Day 2 … list what you want to receive (love, recognition, payment, kindness and so on.)

CHOOSE TO BE HEALTHY

Day 1 – Today I am grateful for all my many blessings.

Day 2 – Today and every day I give what I want to receive.

Day 3 – Today I see all the abundance that surrounds me.

Day 4 – Today I focus on the abundance I want to attract into my life.

Day 5 – Today I accept the abundance flowing to me with thanks and joy.

Day 6 – Today I easily share my talents to bring happiness to myself and others.

Day 7 – Today I embrace my potential to be and do anything I dream.

(The Deepak Chopra Center offers a free 21-day meditation challenge along similar lines.)

Meditation and quiet contemplation along with focused breathing helps to reduce daily stress, slow the heartbeat, lower blood pressure and generally calm frazzled nerves. Work at making it a part of your daily healthy lifestyle.

<u>RESOURCES</u>

(These are in no particular order and are the resources I use most often. There are many more to choose from, these are just a guideline.)

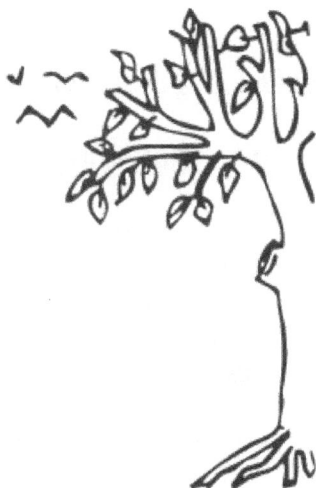

Books

General Health

**Beating Cancer with Nutrition. Patrick Quillan, PhD. (Nutrition Times Press, 2005)
**Diabetes: Tragedy to Triumph. Tracy Herbert. (2016)
**Diet for a New America. John Robbins. (HJ Kramer Books and New World Library,1987)
**Do You Have the Guts to be Beautiful? Jennifer Daniels, MD and Mitra Ray, PhD. (Shining Star Media, 2011)
**Formerly Known as Food. Kristin Lawless. (St. Martin's Press, 2018)
**From Here to Longevity. Mitra Ray, PhD. (Shining Star Publishing, 2004)
**Internal Cleansing. Linda Berry DC. (Three Rivers Press, 2000)
**My Beef With Meat. Rip Esselstyn. (Grand Central Life and Style, 2013)
**Plant Strong. Rip Esselstyn. (Grand Central Life and Style, 2015)
**Raw Energy. Leslie and Susannah Kenton. (Arrow Books Ltd, 1984)
**Seeds of Deception. Jeffery M Smith. (Yes Books, 2003)
**Sports Success Rx. Paul R Stricker, MD, FAAP. (American Academy of Pediatrics Press, 2006)
**The China Study. T Colin Campbell PhD, Thomas M Campbell. (BenBella Books, 2006)
**The Engine 2 Diet. Rip Esselstyn. (Wellness Central, 2009)
**The Healing Foods. Patricia Hausman and Judith Benn Hurley. (Dell Publishing, 1989)
**The Healing Secrets of Food. Deborah Kesten. (New World Library, 2001)
**The NDD Book. (Nutrition Deficit Disorder.) William Sears, MD. (Little, Brown and Company, 2009)
**The Omnivore's Dilemma. Michael Pollan. (Penguin Books, 2006)

**Travel Balance: A unique health guide for your journey. John Ayo. (CreateSpace Independent Publishing, 2017)
**Wheat Belly. Dr William Davies, MD. (Harper Collins Publishers, 2016)
**You are What you Eat. Dr. Gillian McKeith, PhD. (Celador Productions, 2005)
**Your Body Speaks Your Body Heals. Humbart "Smokey" Santillo, ND. (Designs for Wellness Press, 2009)

Juice Plus+® Research

**Juice Plus+®: Clinical Research Quick Reference Guide (4/2018)
**Oxidative Stress in the Pathogenesis of Disease and Aging: Opportunity for Intervention. Richard E. DuBois, MD, FACP. (1998)

Whole Food and Vegan or Vegetarian Recipe Books

**Five-a-Day Fruit and Vegetable Cookbook. Kate Whiteman, Maggie Mayhew and Christine Ingram. (Hermes House, 2007)
**Happy Days with the Naked Chef. Jamie Oliver. (Hyperion Books, 2002)
**Laurel's Kitchen Recipes. Carol Lee flinders, Laurel Robertson, Carol L. Flinders et al. (Ten Speed Press, 2004)
**Plenty. Yottam Ottolenghi. Chronicle Books (2011)
**Rainbow Cuisine. Lannice Snyman and Andrzej Sawa. (S and S Publishers, 1998)

Magazines
Breathe
What Doctors Don't Tell You
Natural Awakenings
Yoga
Reiki
Eat This Not That

Websites

www.taylers.juiceplus.com
www.jamieoliver.com
www.jamiemagazine.com
www.drmitraray.com
www.grainstorm.com
www.thesneakychef.com
www.healthline.com/nutrition
http://gentleworld.org/10-protein-packed-plants
"Top 50 Blogs and Wholefoods Websites to Follow"
www.chopra.com
www.onegreenplanet.org
www.eatthis.com/foods-most-pesticides
www.ehn.org/worst-foods-for-pesticides
www.wddty.com (What Doctors Don't Tell You)
www.mercola.com
No-track Browser: 'DuckDuckGo'

Videos/Movies

The Game Changers – Rip Esselstyn
Forks Over Knives – Rip Esselstyn
Supersize Me – Morgan Spurlock
Fat, Sick and Nearly Dead – Joe Cross
Hungry for Change - James Colquhoun, Laurentine ten Bosch and Mark Hyman
The Man Who Planted Trees - Jean Giono and Jean Roberts 1987 - an animated, heartwarming masterpiece showing what one determined, focused French shepherd accomplished over 30 years.

About the Author

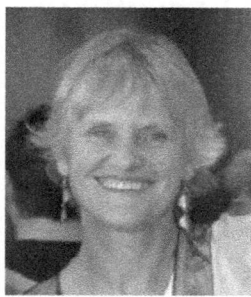

Dr Janet Tayler is a South African native who immigrated to the USA with her husband, Garth, in1995. She is a Naturopath (ND) and is Board Certified in Integrative Medicine. She also holds a BA in Physical Education and an MA in Psychology. She practices from her home in Weatherford, TX

Dr. Tayler has over 30 years of experience as an educator, counselor, speaker, exercise and yoga instructor. As a Doctor of Natural Health, she is on a mission to create awareness of the power of preventative health. She regards most of our so-called "Dread Diseases" as symptoms, even side effects, of our unhealthy and unviable lifestyles.

She believes that carefully-considered nutrition should be a vital part of daily life and is the best way to stay healthy or regain good health. In her view, empowerment, through self-education, is the most cost effective form of health insurance available.

Therapies offered:
Nutrition Counseling   Magnetic Resonancing
Reiki   Reflexology
Stress Management
Yoga postures and Breathing exercises
Independent Juice Plus+® Partner

Available as a Speaker

Contact: janettayler@att.net
Websites: www.tayler.juiceplus.com
    www.holistic-healthpractice.com

Book Janet for Your Next Event

Book Janet as a Speaker or Workshop Facilitator

Most popular topics are in the areas of:
- **Children's Health**
- **Women's Issues**
- **Weight Management**
- **Workplace Health**
- **Family Health**

Some previous presentations have included:
- *"Children's Health: a Non-Negotiable"*
- *"The Recipe for Better Health"*
- *"New Year New You: Your Health in Your Hands."*
- *"Stress the Silent Killer."*
- *"Dem Bones: Osteoporosis Revealed."*
- *Reducing Stress and Hormone Imbalance."*
- *"Heart Health: In Honor of Heart Month."*
- *"Foods that Harm, Foods that Heal.*

Customized presentations and workshops on request.

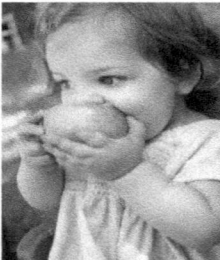

Children's Health

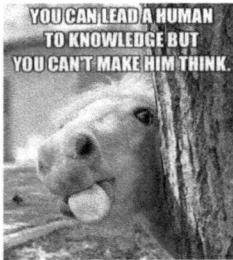

YOU CAN LEAD A HUMAN TO KNOWLEDGE BUT YOU CAN'T MAKE HIM THINK.

Creating Awareness

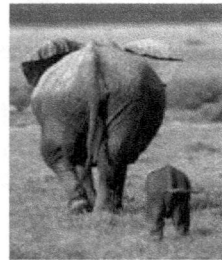

Family Health

<u>Contact</u>:   janettayler@att.net
<u>Websites</u>: www.tayler.juiceplus.com
         www.holistic-healthpractice.com

www.ingramcontent.com/pod-product-compliance
Lightning Source LLC
Chambersburg PA
CBHW022335280326
41934CB00006B/648